D1298875

THE CHILDREN OF CRAIG-Y-NOS

LIFE IN A WELSH TUBERCULOSIS SANATORIUM 1922 – 1959

First published by the Wellcome Trust Centre for the History of Medicine at UCL, 2009

This book is freely available online following the links to Publications at www.ucl.ac.uk/histmed

Book design by Marc Riley, IdeasandCoffee Limited (www.ideasandcoffee.com)
Printed and bound in Great Britain by Lightning Source UK Limited, Milton Keynes

ISBN-10: 0-85484-126-1
ISBN-13: 978-0-85484-126-4

To my late mother,
Marianne Rumsey,
who never missed
a visit in four years.

Ann Shaw

Contents

Acknowledgements

Many people deserve our thanks for making this book possible. First and foremost are those who contributed the stories and photographs, making this a unique and important community project. They have all been extraordinarily supportive, generously giving their time and lending treasured photographs and memorabilia. Malcolm Shaw has been a dedicated supporter since the start of the project and took on the formidable task of digitising over 1200 photographs, of which several hundred are reproduced here. Three photographic collections deserve special mention, those of Christine Perry (Bennett), Mari Friend (Jenkins), and Barbara Pye (Dommett). Brecon Museum, Powys Archives, the Llyfrgell Genedlaethol Cymru/National Library of Wales and Wellcome Images provided additional pictures. Thanks are also due to David and Doreen Rumsey, Ann's brother and sister-in-law, who for decades kept all her photographs of Craig-y-nos, to Karen Howard for support and encouragement, and to Andrew Allan who designed The Children of Craig-y-nos online exhibition (http://childrenofcraigynos.com). Cynthia Mullen and her colleagues at the Sleeping Giant Foundation, Abercraf, conducted interviews in Wales and also liaised with community organisations. Local historian, Len Ley, has always been available for guided tours around Craig-y-nos Castle and unselfishly gave us much of his own research material for inclusion in the book. Valerie Brent (Price), Roy Harry, Valerie Filby, Beryl Richards (Rowlands), Betty Thomas (Dowdle) and Caroline Boyce (Havard) have conducted interviews, been interviewed countless times by the media, mounted and taken down exhibitions, and helped in numerous ways throughout the project. Caroline and Paul Boyce also typed up interviews as did Joan Hamilton, for little financial reward.

We are indebted to staff at the Miners' Welfare and Community Hall, Ystradgynlais, Brecon Library, and Swansea Museum, for holding the photographic exhibitions that have been so successful and engendered such a keen interest in 'The Children of Craig-y-nos'. Similarly, staff at Craig-y-nos Castle have been enormously accommodating and enthusiastic supporters, and we cannot imagine a more exciting place from which to launch the book. Support for Carole Reeves has come from the Wellcome Trust Centre for the History of Medicine, University College London, and she particularly wishes to thank Professor Anne Hardy, Professor Hal Cook and Alan Shiel. Carole also wishes to acknowledge her late father, George Reeves, for love and enthusiasm for a project close to his own heart although, sadly, he did not live to see the publication of this book. The Llyfrgell Genedlaethol Cymru/National Library of Wales, Powys Archives, National Archives, and Wellcome Library, London, have been important sources of information to contextualise the oral histories and provide the historical framework on which to construct the 'missing' history of Craig-y-nos. We realise, in the absence of hospital records that much may still be missing but hope that the best possible compromise has been reached and that the book offers new insights into the sanatorium experience of young people with tuberculosis in Wales. The Welsh media has been hugely supportive of the project since it began and we are grateful to the moderators of the BBC Mid Wales community history website, BBC Radio Wales, S4C, *South Wales Evening Post*, *Brecon and Radnor Express* and 0639 Community Magazine. Finally, our immense gratitude to the Big Lottery Fund – Awards for All Wales, without whose generous grant this book would not have been published.

Preface

Clive Rowlands - I kicked a rugby ball through the glass door

I was admitted to Craig-y-nos as an eight-year-old, in 1947. That winter was the snowiest since 1814 and among the coldest on record, but our beds were wheeled out onto the balcony so that our lungs would benefit from the sharp, icy mountain air. A nurse would take a few of us for a walk in the grounds to the lake and point out animal footprints in the snow.

Although I was one of five children, I don't think I suffered as much as other youngsters from separation from my family because my sister, in her early twenties, was already in Craig-y-nos and I was allowed to see her every day. I also benefited from her weekly visitors because children's visiting was normally only once a month. However, I wasn't aware that my sister was terminally ill and she was later sent home to die. I remember the gastric lavages – horrible – and still shudder when I recall the coldness of X-ray plates against my chest. Of the staff, I remember Matron Knox-Thomas, Dr Jordan – a lovely doctor – and Dr Hubbard who walked with a limp – the kind of thing that stays in a child's mind. My most abiding memory, however, is of receiving the gift of a rugby ball from Elwyn Dewi Hopkins, a lad from my home village of Cwmtwrch, and being punished for kicking it through a glass door. I was put in a straitjacket for a week.

After a year in Craig-y-nos, I was sent for rehabilitation to Highland Moors, an institution for convalescent boys in the mid-Wales spa town of Llandrindod Wells, which was like a public school compared with the strict sanatorium regime. At Highland Moors, the emphasis was on outdoor activities and fitness and I spent hours playing football, which helped to lay the groundwork for my subsequent sporting career. When I came home to my village of Cwmtwrch I was the only one there not wearing a vest! By the time I left Highland Moors I was not only physically fit and very sporty but mature beyond my years. I was used to making my own decisions. I had become a leader.

Clive Rowlands, OBE
Former captain and coach of the Welsh Rugby team
Manager, British and Irish Lions tour to Australia, 1989
Manager, British Isles team v a rest of the world team, 1986
Manager, Wales in the Rugby World Cup, 1987
President of the Welsh Rugby Union, 1989

Introduction

Craig-y-nos, meaning 'rock of the night', is the name of a hill that rises above the Tawe valley on the south-west edge of the Brecon Beacons National Park. The country house, which is adjacent to it and took its name, was built in 1840 by Captain Rice Davies Powell, member of a local landowning family. Below a steep bank at the rear of the house flowed the River Tawe in its journey south to the sea at Abertawe (Swansea) twenty-three miles away, whilst passing the front door was the recently completed road between the market town of Ystradgynlais and the city of Brecon. Powell died in 1862, having been predeceased by his wife and two of his four children. Within a couple of years, his heir had been killed in a hunting accident and his remaining daughter, Sarah, lived on the estate with her husband, Captain Allaway. After Allaway's death, the estate was sold in 1876 to Morgan Morgan, a gentleman of Ystradgynlais, for £7000, but due to financial difficulties, the family was obliged to sell just two years later for half the purchase price.

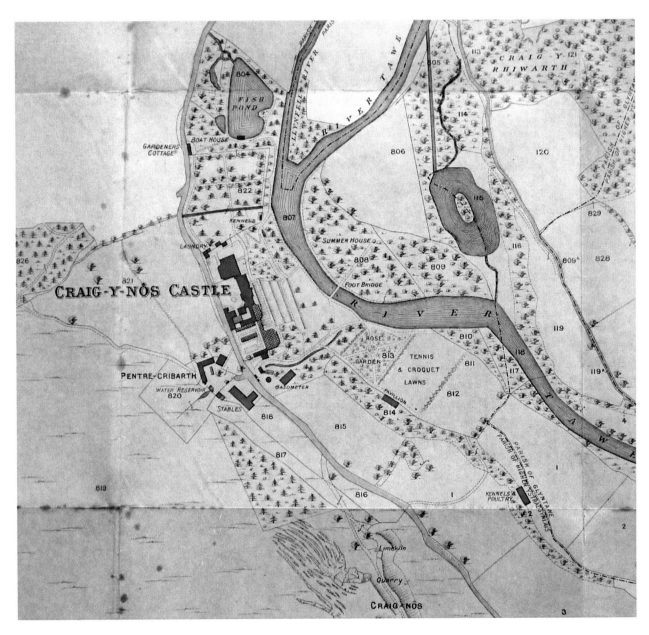

Map of Craig-y-nos estate, c.1900. In Craig-y-nos Castle estate brochure, 1901. Courtesy Llyfrgell Genedlaethol Cymru/National Library of Wales.

The new owner of the seventeen-acre estate was Adelina Patti (1843-1919), the world famous Italian-born opera singer, who spent over £100,000 laying out and extending the grounds and house (the term 'castle' seems to have arrived with Patti), adding the north and south wings, clock tower, conservatory, hot houses, magnificent winter garden, and theatre – now a Grade-I listed building. Patti was one of the highest paid performers of the age. A tour of South America in 1889, for example, earned over £100,000 in fees (£1250 a night), and she commanded $5000 a performance during her 1883 tour of the United States. Patti's career was long and successful. Her first season at London's Covent Garden was in 1861 and her final professional concert was at the Albert Hall, London, in 1906. Although renowned as a hard bargainer in the professional world of opera, Patti was kind to her staff and generous to communities around Craig-y-nos, raising hundreds of pounds for local hospitals through charity concerts. The estate was an important source of employment for people living several miles from the collieries and iron works in the lower Tawe valley, and the oral testimonies of Phil Lewis and Ken Lewis evoke some of the atmosphere of the community when Patti was presiding as 'lady bountiful'. By 1900, she employed more than forty domestic staff and up to thirty estate workers, and in addition, all the furniture and furnishings of the castle were manufactured to Patti's order by a company (B Evans & Co) in Swansea. Craig-y-nos was one of the first private houses in Britain to be fitted with electric lighting, the electricity being generated by an 'Otto' gas engine fuelled from a small gas works in the grounds (see estate map). Guests from all over the world, including British and foreign royalty, were entertained at Craig-y-nos, and Patti's own extensive travels began and ended at the isolated railway station in the village of Penwyllt, overlooking the castle, where a small but richly furnished waiting room was placed at her disposal. The railway company provided a locomotive to pull her sumptuously appointed private railway carriage, and in 1887, she opened the Severn Tunnel, which carried a new railway between London and Neath.

Patti's importance and generosity to the communities of South Wales were recognised by the local honours bestowed upon her, the most prestigious being the freedom of the cities of Brecon (1897) and Swansea (1912).[1] By the people of the Tawe valley, a number of whose ancestors were employed at Craig-y-nos, she is still respectfully referred to as Madame Patti. Phil Lewis's cousin, Betty Lewis, who was born in 1908 and became a ward sister at Craig-y-nos in the mid-1950s, recalled the enthusiastic crowds that always followed Patti's local excursions despite her long residence in the community. Betty's uncle, David Hughes, was the incumbent at Callwen's Church, Glyntawe, and acted as Patti's chaplain,[2] and later as chaplain to the sanatorium.[3]

Patti died on 27 September 1919, and in March 1921, her third husband, Baron Olaf Rudolph Cederström, sold – for £19,000 – the entire estate of forty-eight acres to the King Edward VII Welsh National Memorial Association (WNMA).[4] The WNMA was established in 1910 (and granted a Royal Charter in 1912) with a particular remit to prevent, treat and eradicate tuberculosis (TB) in Wales.[5] It began by raising over £300,000 through voluntary subscriptions, half of which was contributed by its first president, David Davies, MP, later Lord Davies of Llandinam (1880-1944). The money was spent on initiating an educational campaign and in providing hospitals and sanatoria. Provision was made for a hospital at Swansea and a site (at Singleton) was acquired. However, owing to the very high building costs after the First World War (1914-18), the scheme was abandoned in favour of the acquisition and adaptation of Craig-y-nos Castle to a 100-bed sanatorium, named the Adelina Patti Hospital.[6] In the same year (1921), the Public Health (Tuberculosis) Act made it obligatory for all the county councils and county borough councils of Wales to provide treatment for people with tuberculosis. Each council entrusted the WNMA with this task and levied a community tax to pay for it.[7] By 1930, the WNMA had provided sixteen hospitals and sanatoria in Wales, together with some 100 dispensaries and clinics. Its capital expenditure was £500,000, half of which came from voluntary funds and the remainder from central and local government grants.[8] The WNMA was disbanded in 1948 at the inauguration of the National Health Service (NHS), by which time it funded 2600 beds, seventy doctors, 580 nursing and 830 domestic staff, a mobile mass X-ray unit, a research laboratory and a Chair of Tuberculosis at the Welsh National School of Medicine, Cardiff.[9]

Tuberculosis is a very ancient infectious disease caused by a bacterium. Both humans and animals can catch TB but the strains of bacteria are different. Bioarchaeologists at University College London and Tel-Aviv University have recently discovered TB in the remains of a mother and her baby in Israel, which are 9000 years old. They lived at the time when humans were beginning to settle in agricultural communities but before dairy farming. This challenges the long-held belief that human TB evolved from bovine TB, a disease of cattle (most of our infectious diseases seem to have been passed to us from domesticated animals in pre-historic times).[10] Although the human strain of TB bacteria is older by 3000 thousand years than was previously thought, it was only discovered in 1882 by a German bacteriologist, Robert Koch. Koch named it *Mycobacterium tuberculosis*. The only animal tuberculosis able to infect humans is *Mycobacterium bovis*, which is usually transmitted by ingesting infected milk or meat. Bovine TB has always been more of a problem in children than adults. By 1931, for example, over 1000 children in England and Wales were dying from bovine TB each year. During the 1930s, tuberculin testing (for TB) was introduced in British cattle, and forty per cent were found to be reactors. Pasteurisation, introduced initially to preserve milk, helped control the transmission of bovine disease to humans, although it was 1960 before all British milk was required to be pasteurised.

Although TB bacteria can cause disease in any part of the body, it is mainly transmitted through the air during talking, coughing and sneezing. This is why the lungs are most commonly infected. Epidemics of tuberculosis have often occurred at times of urbanisation because it is associated with poor and overcrowded living conditions. There was also an association during the Industrial Revolution with occupations such as coal and tin mining, iron smelting, textile production, and pottery manufacture. Tuberculosis killed more people during the nineteenth century than any other disease. Thirteen per cent of all deaths in England and Wales from 1851 to 1910 were from TB, but of young adults aged twenty to twenty-four, almost half died of the disease. Consumption (TB of the lungs) accounted for sixty to eighty per cent of all tuberculosis deaths. It claimed a larger proportion of women's than men's lives, partly because of pregnancy and inferior nutrition in cases where working men in poor households were given the best food. The sanatorium movement, based on open-air treatment and education in self-care, was well established by the beginning of the twentieth century but survival was generally poor. For example, of the 3000 patients discharged in 1927 from sanatoria run by the London County Council, only twenty-four per cent were still alive by 1932.[11]

The Adelina Patti Hospital – more commonly known as Craig-y-nos – admitted tuberculosis patients from 1922 until 1959 when it became an eighty-bed hospital for the chronically sick, most particularly those with chronic chest diseases such as pneumoconiosis, silicosis and bronchitis. These conditions were related to coal mining, slate quarrying, and other dust-laden Welsh industries. By 1962, Craig-y-nos was largely a geriatric hospital and threatened with closure due to the proposed new district general hospital at Singleton Park, Swansea, destined to have a bed capacity of 500 to 800, serving a population of 150,000. However, there was much concern in the rural area around Craig-y-nos about loss of jobs (the hospital employed 109 staff) in an area of high unemployment.[12] A mass protest against closure in 1968 drew not only on its importance as an employer but on its history as the home of Adelina Patti. An emotionally-laden petition spoke for its 6000 signatories: 'Take away the hospital and Madame Patti's association will fade into oblivion. We cannot afford such a loss. Our only monuments will be coal and slag tips.' Despite the retort of the Welsh Hospital Board that attractive old buildings did not provide accommodation in accordance with modern hospital concepts,[13] Craig-y-nos remained open until 1986. Its final patients were transferred to a new Community Hospital at Ystradgynlais and the building was put up for sale by auction.[14] The castle's present owner purchased it in 2000, and converted it to a hotel and conference centre although renovations and restorations are ongoing. The castle's splendid façade and rare Grade-1 listed theatre, original interior features and location, make it an ideal venue for weddings. Organised 'ghost hunts' exploit the legend that Adelina Patti's ghost still haunts the castle and grounds.

The 'Children of Craig-y-nos' project was begun in 2006 by Ann Shaw who visited Craig-y-nos Castle with her husband, Malcolm, for the first time in over fifty years. Curiosity had brought her back to see the place where she had spent four years (1950-54) as a child with tuberculosis, perhaps seeking some kind of closure. A member of the hotel staff who had shown them around the dilapidated old wards told her that all the records of its time as a hospital had been destroyed, but that occasionally ex-patients turned up seeking information. Just the previous week, for example, Roy Harry had made *his* first visit since leaving as a five-year-old in 1946. He and Ann, quite independently, had been thinking about their experiences at Craig-y-nos and been drawn back to the old mansion. Ann launched a blog (www.craig-y-nos.blogspot.com) in November 2006 to find other ex-patients and to collect their memories of Craig-y-nos with a view to publishing them as a book. Then, in April 2007, Sylvia Moore (Peckham), who had been both a patient and a nurse, organised the first ever reunion, which was attended by about sixty people, mostly ex members of staff. Clearly, there was a budding collective interest in the hospital's history. When Ann returned to her home in Scotland she searched the internet in vain for information about the castle's decades as a TB sanatorium but found Carole Reeves, who had just been appointed to the post of outreach historian at the Wellcome Trust Centre for the History of Medicine, University College London. Carole confirmed that there were, indeed, no known hospital records but was intrigued to know more, not least because her mother had been born and raised near this area of South Wales, into a family that had experienced the cold touch of tuberculosis.

Ann and Carole sat at opposite ends of Britain staring into the same void – forty years of missing Welsh history. What to do? Ann put her thoughts onto the BBC Mid Wales community history website: 'Part of me says, why dig up the past? Why resurrect memories best buried and forgotten? The bad old days are over. TB is no longer a killer. There are miracle drugs. Yet I sense a need for closure, not just for myself but for all the people who are still alive, and their families too, for TB affected the whole community, not just physically but socially and emotionally. It was the disease never spoken about except in hushed whispers. Craig-y-nos was called a hospital but it had all the hallmarks of a prison for sick children. It was isolated and resembled an impenetrable fortress. Cars were almost non-existent and transport consisted of the local train and an infrequent bus service provided by the South Wales Transport and Western Welsh bus companies. On visiting days, these also organised special coaches to pick up visitors at designated stopping places throughout South Wales. The average length of stay was two to three years and on arrival you were stripped of most possessions.

A few years ago, I was visiting my father in a residential home in Crickhowell and a ninety-year-old woman asked me who I was. I reverted to the Welsh rural practice of identifying myself by name and the farm I come from: Ann – Ty-Llangenny. Without a moment's hesitation, she replied, "You are the one who was very ill." We have long memories in Wales.'

And so it turned out. No sooner had Ann posted these comments on her blog and put an appeal in the *South Wales Evening Post* than the stories, photographs and telephone calls began flooding in from all over the UK, and many parts of the world, especially the USA, Canada, Australia and New Zealand. There is no doubt that the internet has made this project possible. Within seven months, with the help of Cynthia Mullen and the Sleeping Giant Foundation, ex-nurse Valerie Brent (Price) and ex-patient Caroline Boyce (Havard), the project had collected over eighty written and oral testimonies and other scrupulously preserved memorabilia, and an incredible collection of 600 photographs, mostly taken by the children themselves on simple box cameras. These photographs, taken between fifty and eighty-five years ago, gave a unique insight into life inside a TB sanatorium. Not as a daily record of events but as a most evocative revelation of youthful stoicism and zest for life at a time when TB in South Wales claimed the lives of twelve young men and seventeen young women a year in every community of 6000 people. Hundreds of others, like the children of Craig-y-nos, were deprived by chronic ill health of education, work and family life.

The first photographic exhibition was held in September 2007 at the Miners' Welfare and Community Hall, Ystradgynlais, seven miles from Craig-y-nos. To coincide with its launch, a reunion for ex-patients and staff took place on Sunday 9 September at the castle and was attended by over 120 people. For some such as Mary Davies (Morris) it was their first visit to the castle since they had left as children, and it proved an extremely emotional experience. Others, living locally, had made regular visits to walk in the grounds, which in 1976 became a country park. A number, out of curiosity, became reacquainted with the estate when the project began, slipping back quietly to look for familiar marks on the exterior walls remembered from years on the balconies; to search for a lost childhood. Local historian, Len Ley, spent much time on that Sunday giving guided tours of the castle's upper floors where the fixtures, fittings and layout of the old wards, though much decayed, were still in evidence so that people were able to recognise their particular bed spaces. In November, the exhibition moved to Brecon Library where it remained until January 2008. By this time the project had collected many more stories and a further 600 photographs. For Malcolm Shaw, the work of digitising and cataloguing these became almost a full-time job. Ann's original objective, to incorporate the oral testimonies and photographs into a book, was given impetus in March 2008 when the Big Lottery Fund, under the Awards for All Wales scheme, awarded £5000 to University College London for Ann and Carole to produce a print-on-demand publication. This, in turn, paved the way for a third exhibition at Swansea Museum during the summer of 2008. The Museum became a meeting place for many ex-patients. They often joined Valerie Brent (Price), a nurse at Craig-y-nos from 1945 to 1947, who 'manned' the exhibition for two days each week and delighted in talking to visitors of all ages. It was largely due to the community volunteers that over 600 people from around the world signed the exhibition's visitors' book. In addition, BBC Radio Wales produced a thirty-minute documentary entitled 'Bed Rest, Pine Trees and Fresh Air: Welsh Sanatoria', transmitted on 31 August 2008, which featured interviews with Carole, Roy, Valerie and Betty Thomas (Dowdle).

As far as we are aware, this is the first ever collective account by patients and staff of life inside a tuberculosis sanatorium and is therefore an historical project of some significance. There is a growing interest in the effects of long-term hospitalisation of children, and the TB experience is central to this because it is the only illness that kept children in hospital for years on end. (The institutions for children with learning difficulties served a different purpose and much has been written about them). There are a few recent studies of childhood tuberculosis and sanatoria including an autobiographical account by Rosemary Conry of her three years in Cappagh Hospital near Dublin,[15] a doctoral thesis by Susan Kelly on childhood TB in Northern Ireland for which she interviewed fifty-three ex-patients,[16] and an American study of the tuberculosis 'preventorium', an institution for children considered at risk of TB.[17] Although the Craig-y-nos hospital records and case notes are not available, there are other records that shed light on its management, day to day activities and the lives of its patients and staff. These include the surviving records of the Welsh National Memorial Association, Records of the Ministry of Education (school inspectors' reports), Records of the Welsh Office, the Welsh Hospital Board and the General Nursing Council for England and Wales (hospital inspectors' reports). In addition, contemporary articles in newspapers and medical journals, pamphlets and books, provide essential information about the cultural and scientific environment in which Craig-y-nos operated alongside many other tuberculosis institutions.

This book contains the stories of over ninety people who were children, teenagers, young adults and staff at Craig-y-nos, or who had relatives there. In this sense, it is a community oral history project and not a work of academic research. Although we did not initially set out to draw conclusions about the long-term effects of admission to this sanatorium with its attendant deprivation of family and community life, certain patterns have emerged. John Bowlby, the influential child psychiatrist who was one of the first, in the 1940s and 1950s, to highlight emotional disturbances in children separated from their parents at a young age, considered children with tuberculosis to be a special case. Very many, he noted, came from families where other members, especially parents, had tuberculosis (by whom they had been infected) so that illness and death were common. There was much disruption and anxiety in these families, which was an additional burden to the separation caused by admission for a prolonged period of time to a sanatorium. Also, many children had been separated from their families in a succession of other hospitals prior to the sanatorium experience.[18] These observations hold true for the children and young people admitted to Craig-y-nos, of whom twenty-four had witnessed parents, siblings and other family members suffering or dying from tuberculosis. In some cases, the death of a parent occurred immediately prior to the child's admission, which in effect resulted also in the loss of the surviving parent. Those who seem to have been most adversely affected by the Craig-y-nos experience were admitted as pre-school children, or before the age of five, when the mother-child relationship is at a critical stage in the child's social development. They talk of becoming 'self-reliant', 'a loner', 'tough as nails' and 'independent', traits common in children who seem to become well adjusted to their hospital surroundings but who develop what is considered to be an abnormal indifference or detachment from their mothers which spills over into an inability to make relationships in later life. Experts today, such as child psychiatrist, Professor Sir Michael Rutter, do not place the same emphasis as Bowlby on the mother as the all-important figure in a child's early life. Professor Rutter argues that most children, throughout history, have formed multiple attachments to those with whom they have had close continuous contact such as grandparents, aunts, uncles, and carers, etc. So the separation, whilst important, may not be as disruptive and psychologically damaging to the child as that of a severely malfunctioning family.[19] Indeed, when Bowlby followed up young people who had been admitted to a sanatorium as very young children, he was surprised to find how well adjusted most of them seemed to be.

Nevertheless, in the case of Craig-y-nos, it is the people who were admitted as older children and teenagers who recall the most positive memories. For a few such as Sylvia Moore (Peckham), whose parents were divorced and Christine Perry (Bennett), who was brought up by her grandparents, it is remembered as one of the happiest periods of their lives. Others were not so enthusiastic but made the best of it. Some, however, found it a distressing experience, and even at a distance of fifty or sixty years, broke down when reliving deeply buried memories. Some were unable to talk at all but communicated entirely though e.mail. A few remember physical and sexual abuse by staff. Face-slapping by teachers and similar chastisement, which today would constitute abuse, was considered acceptable corporal punishment during the hospital decades. Use of restraint by tying children to cot and bed railings with tapes stitched to clothing (called straitjackets by ex-patients) was justified by over-stretched staff but criticized by hospital inspectors. Even keeping five-year-olds in high-sided cots, as was the norm in the babies' ward, could be interpreted as a form of imprisonment. The physical isolation of Craig-y-nos was another. Only one young woman, Eileen Gibbons (Hill), admits to successful escape although several teenagers and children made abortive bids for freedom. Eileen's walk-out was a very brave act given that patients were warned that self-discharge would result in being 'written off' by the medical authorities. In other words, they could not expect to be treated if their tuberculosis returned. That so few left Craig-y-nos of their own volition is remarkable because self-discharge from British sanatoria was not uncommon. West Wales Sanatorium (Llanybyther), for example, was notorious during the 1920s and 1930s for its inability to keep patients. It had received such bad press publicity that many parents, according to Dr Charles Lloyd, the Tuberculosis Officer for Cardiganshire, likened it to a reformatory for children rather than a sanatorium.[20] Even after patients had been officially discharged from sanatoria, they were often followed up for decades, which caused embarrassment and resentment among those aiming to keep their medical histories a secret from friends, colleagues and employers. Betty Thomas (Dowdle), who left Llanybyther Sanatorium in 1942, maintained that 'No one would employ you if you said that you had TB', but later, in the 1950s, when TB was considered 'curable' by antibiotics, employment discrimination seems to have been less of an issue. Pat Hybert (Mogridge) returned to work in her old office in 1953, and Barbara O'Connell (Paines) worked in a factory where, if she had a 'bad day', her bosses would be sympathetic and give her the 'easy jobs'. Some ex-patients such as Barbara Pye (Dommett), Rosemary Davies (Harley), and Mary Watkins (Williams) opted to work outside in the open air whilst others, like Haydn Beynon and Alan Morgan became coal miners and steel workers, occupations associated with increased rates of TB and other chest diseases.

Women but not men recollect the patronising attitudes of clinic staff, after discharge from the sanatorium, from whom they were obliged to seek permission before performing daily tasks such as hair washing, and returning to work. Again, it is the women who report having to gain permission to marry and start a family. Barbara Pye (Dommett) was given the all-clear five years after she left Craig-y-nos. Others, like Carol Hughes (Davies) were less compliant and had their children without asking permission. The disturbing experience of Betty Thomas (Dowdle) who, in 1945, was forced to have an abortion at five months pregnant, is in stark contrast to Olive Pamela Joseph, whose last three children (she already had two children when she was admitted to Craig-y-nos) were born in quick succession with the blessing of the clinic doctor. The fifteen-year period between these two experiences coincided, not only with changing attitudes towards the curability of tuberculosis but also in ideas about its hereditary nature. By the late 1950s, only the most unenlightened medical professionals still clung to the notion of it being passed down genetically from mother to child. Nevertheless, there is a suggestion among experts today that what some individuals may inherit is a susceptibility to tuberculosis, perhaps by having a genetically weaker ability to acquire immunity. They argue that natural selection weeds out highly susceptible individuals either by killing them (through TB) or restricting the number of children they produce. Part of the current increase in tuberculosis, they suggest, may be caused by effective drug treatment eliminating natural selection.[21] The comment made by the Committee of Enquiry into the Anti-tuberculosis Service in Wales in 1937, that 'families are either free from the disease or riddled with it',[22] is an observation that can be endorsed by the stories from Craig-y-nos. Certainly, the tuberculosis infection did leave many women unable to have children. In the Welsh culture, which is very family-orientated, this caused distress to a number of the ex-patients of Craig-y-nos for whom adoption was not possible because of their history of tuberculosis. One who circumvented this was Lynette Davies (Evans), whose infection damaged her fallopian tubes but who adopted two children by the simple expedient of not informing the adoption authorities of her past tuberculosis: 'They never asked so I never told them.' Eileen Gibbons (Hill) became a foster mother after losing three little boys.

There is often a tendency in collective remembrance to romanticise the past and to moderate its dark side. We have observed that the more reunions that have taken place between ex-patients and between ex-patients and staff, the more moderated these memories have become. Importantly, some of the anger clearly present in early conversations has been de-fused by the process of working through shared memories. The daily blog, set up by Ann Shaw at the end of 2006, has been the posting board for stories revised two, three and four times over. Which are the 'real' ones? Who can tell. The majority of the interviews in this book were conducted between January and October 2007, prior to most of the reunions, and on a one-to-one basis. All but one of the forty interviews conducted by Carole Reeves, were recorded over the telephone. Telephone interviews have advantages and disadvantages. Lack of personal contact may inhibit some interviewees but others prefer the telephone's anonymity, and talking to an empathetic stranger presents few problems. In any case, and importantly, the oral testimonies contain only those memories that the interviewees were prepared to share at the time of interview. Ann Shaw's 100-plus interviews (not all are included in the book but most are on the blog) are a mix of those conducted on the telephone and those gathered on her visits to Wales. Interviews by Valerie Brent, by oral historians at the Sleeping Giant Foundation, and other community volunteers, were individually collected, usually in the interviewees' homes. Telephone interviews were conducted by Caroline Boyce (Havard), who now lives in Scotland. Transcribed interviews were sent to interviewees for agreement and in some cases, additional material has been added from follow-up conversations and letters. All those whose edited interviews are included in the book have signed a form giving permission for their memories to be published and for the tapes, copies of their photographs, and other memorabilia to be placed in the Powys Archives, Llandrindod Wells.

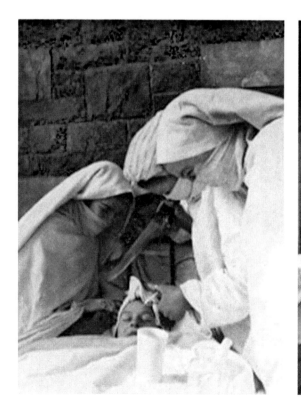

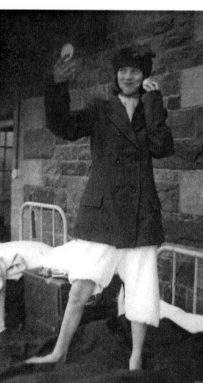

A realistic re-enactment of an operation by children in Ward 2. The threat of lung surgery, ever present and always dreaded, was part of the distress of TB. Courtesy Ann Shaw.

Christine Perry (Bennett) recalls a happy three years in Craig-y-nos despite having a number of relapses. Courtesy Christine Perry.

As a self-selected group, the participants have given us stories that may not, in fact, be wholly representative of the castle's history as a sanatorium. There are, for example, notable gaps in our knowledge of people who were patients in at least three of the main wards. In addition, it will soon become apparent that there are far more oral testimonies from women than men – over three-quarters are from women. We do not know whether this was due to a reticence on the part of men to come forward but there were certainly fewer men than women in Craig-y-nos right up until 1945 when the men were moved out completely. In 1936, for example, there were twice as many girls and women as boys and men.[23] There is also the question of survival. Women's life expectancy is longer than men's so it is reasonable to expect a higher death rate amongst men in the decades between leaving Craig-y-nos and the start of this project. We have no way of knowing how many ex-patients have died due to a resurgence of their tuberculosis, a not uncommon occurrence because *Mycobacterium tuberculosis* may remain dormant in the body for decades, becoming activated when the immune system is weakened by illness or old age (this is known as post-primary infection). Indeed, a number of interviewees have experienced recent reactivation of tuberculosis.

Although this is an historical study, TB is not a disease of history. During the 1960s and 1970s, it appeared to come largely under control but since the mid-1980s there has been a worldwide increase of about one per cent a year. In the United Kingdom, the increase has been nearer to two per cent, although very high rates in London have somewhat skewed the national figures.[24] The World Health Organization in 1993 declared TB a public health emergency and the disease remains a major cause of death worldwide. An estimated 8.8 million people were diagnosed with TB in 2005 and 1.6 million died of it. The highest rates of infection occur in developing and reconstructing countries, beset by wars, homelessness, poor sanitation, poverty and HIV/AIDS. The really serious problem is the worldwide spread of strains of *Mycobacterium tuberculosis* that are resistant to the drugs available to treat TB. Although research teams are working to investigate new drugs and to test existing ones in various permutations, many experts believe that the eventual eradication of tuberculosis will rest on a political commitment to tackle problems of world poverty, inequality and inadequate access to health care.[25]

However difficult it becomes to control tuberculosis both locally and globally, one thing is certain. Those infected will never again be isolated from the rest of society because history has shown that policing infectious diseases is neither workable nor humane. Considering what we now know about the psychological effects of stigmatisation, separation and life-threatening illness, the Children of Craig-y-nos could be a story of destruction or defeat but, indeed, it is one of courage and survival. Despite years of illness and lost education, and given the limited career opportunities in Wales at the time, many went on to achieve success as doctors, nurses, teachers, writers, journalists, artists, college lecturers, accountants and secretaries. Millionaires, mayors, a hospital administrator, a theatre director and an international rugby player emerged from the plaster cast, the collapsed lung and the confinement of Craig-y-nos Castle.

Ann Shaw and Carole Reeves
February 2009

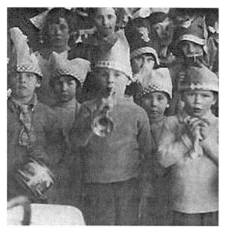
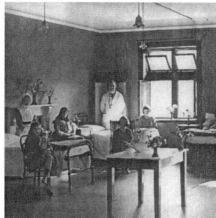
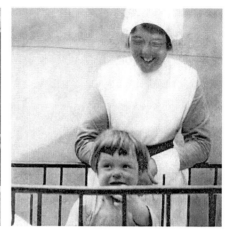

1920s

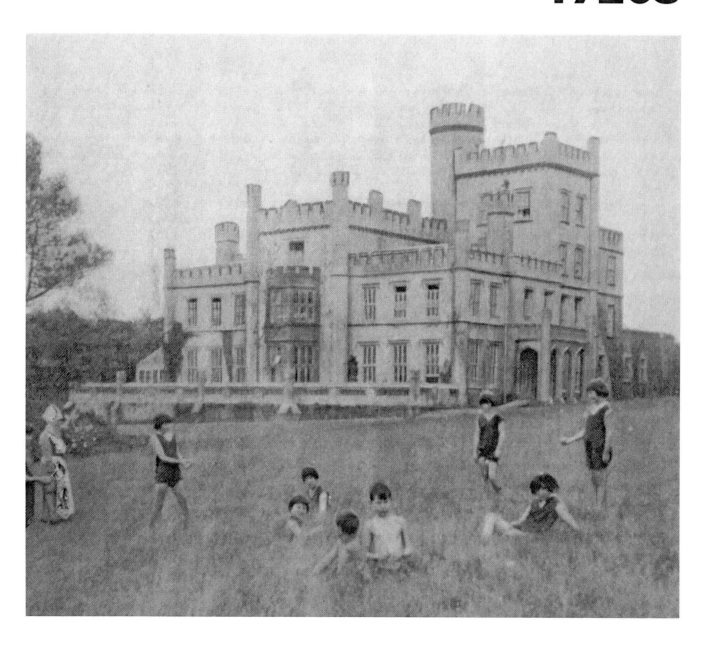

Splendid isolation – Craig-y-nos, TB and treatment in the 1920s

The conversion of Craig-y-nos from a richly appointed private residence to a Spartan sanatorium was accomplished very quickly during the summer and autumn of 1921. The most striking structural alteration was the erection of a cast iron and concrete roofed balcony block attached to the rear of the main house, enabling patients on the ground, first and second floor wards to live outdoors and benefit from the fresh air blowing across the Brecon Beacons. The location of Craig-y-nos, amidst mountains and pine woods was typical of the tuberculosis institutions advocating 'open-air treatment', based on those established in Germany in the late nineteenth century. Particularly influential in this regard was Dr Otto Walther, whose sanatorium built at Nordrach-in-Baden, in the Black Forest, in 1888, was visited by many British doctors, of whom a number went to be cured of tuberculosis themselves.[1] Just six years earlier, another German, Dr Robert Koch, had discovered the tuberculosis germ (*Mycobacterium tuberculosis*), which proved that TB was an infectious disease and not hereditary as previously believed. Despite this revolutionary discovery, the stigma associated with TB remained to haunt its unfortunate sufferers until well into the twentieth century. Welsh poet-physician, Dannie Abse, who worked for many years as a chest specialist, captures in his poem, 'Tuberculosis', the sardonic despair of a recently diagnosed friend:

'TB I've got. You know what TB signifies?
Totally buggered.' He laughed. His sister cried.

Tuberculosis was as much a social disease – associated with poverty, overcrowded living, maternal ignorance, alcoholism, insanity, over-exertion, and 'bad habits' – as it was a medical condition. People who caught the infection often found themselves ostracized because of the social aspects, and isolated because of its infectious nature. Craig-y-nos, like other sanatoria, was located a considerable distance from a population centre. It was well known that local populations objected to sanatoria being established in their immediate vicinities, and some parishes organized petitions opposing such proposals. Robert Koch, who won a Nobel Prize in 1905 for his work on tuberculosis, contributed to its stigmatisation by suggesting, in his Nobel Lecture that as the decline in leprosy had been brought about by the segregation of its afflicted, so the same could be achieved in tuberculosis.[2]

Craig-y-nos opened its doors to patients on 4 August 1922. It admitted men and women with pulmonary (lung) tuberculosis, and children with non-pulmonary infection, that is, TB of the bones and joints, skin, lymph glands, abdomen, etc. Non-pulmonary tuberculosis was much more common in children than adults. The first Medical Superintendent was Dr Frank Wells, who had qualified at St Mary's Hospital, London, in 1911. Other staff appointed in 1921 included Sister Nona Evans who became Matron

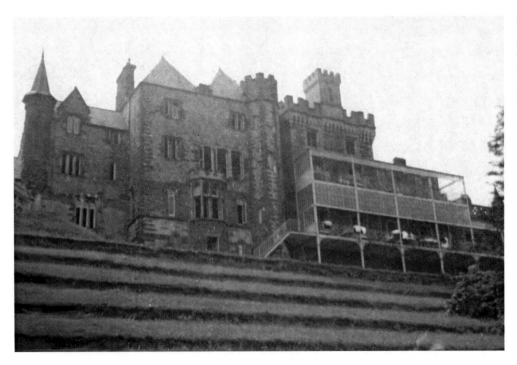

Balconies at Craig-y-nos. These were built when the castle was converted to a sanatorium. They were roofed and the sides were glazed but until the 1950s the fronts were open to the elements. Courtesy Mari Friend.

in 1934, Sister Margaret Phillips, S J Jones, a probationer (student nurse), who stayed until 1925, W Hibbert, a stoker, whose family had been employed by Patti, and Kate Dixon, a nurses' maid who caught tuberculosis and was admitted as a patient to Glan Ely Hospital, Cardiff.[3] Staff were employed by the Welsh National Memorial Association (WNMA) and not by individual sanatoria. As a result, individuals were transferred between sanatoria on temporary and permanent contracts, perhaps from choice and also to cater for staff shortages and sickness. Fifty-eight appointments were made in 1922 including nurses, probationers, ward maids, maids for nurses' and doctors' quarters, cooks, kitchen and laundry staff, gardeners, carpenters, an electrician, a chauffeur and a head porter. Of these appointments, twenty-six resigned within one year of service, an extraordinarily high staff turnover, which must have adversely affected the morale of the new hospital. The lack of consistent staff registers makes it difficult to assess whether this was an ongoing problem but even in 1934, the Medical Superintendent was complaining that most of the probationers appointed during the past six months had left of their own accord.[4] Certainly, the restrictions imposed on young resident female staff (see the oral testimonies of Valerie Brent (Price) and Glenys Jones (Davies)) were uncompromising as illustrated by the case of AT, a probationer appointed in 1924, who received instant dismissal for being caught smoking on the castle roof.[5]

During Patti's residence, the estate grounds had been carefully stocked and managed for shooting and fishing. A large fish pond contained hatching grounds, the lake was well filled with trout, together with excellent trout fishing in the River Tawe, and pheasants, partridges, snipe, duck and other wing and ground game were plentiful.[6] Poaching would surely have occurred then as it most certainly did in the 1920s. In August 1927, a Thomas J Davies was about to be prosecuted by the WNMA for illegally fishing and using illegal bait (salmon roe) until someone had the bright idea of offering him the fishing and shooting rights for five years, for which he paid £30 a year, and held until at least 1947.[7] Thomas Davies appears to have been no ordinary poacher because by 1935 he was Vice-Chairman of the House Committee of the Adelina Patti Hospital! 'Nightlines in the river', the oral testimony of Peter Wagstaffe, reveals that Mr Davies must himself have turned a blind eye to the poaching carried on in the war years by the children to augment the rations of the sickest patients.

Although the full cost of refurbishing the castle as a sanatorium is not known, the total capital expenditure in the first decade amounted to £50,000, half of which came from Exchequer grants and the rest from voluntary contributions.[8] The very first items of equipment purchased for its medical, administrative, household and recreational activities totalled £1418 and included slate slabs for lockers, tennis nets, croquet sets, syringes, measuring standards, bed rests, brushes, preserving pans, alarm clocks, rubber gloves, wooden pattens (slipped over shoes to raise the feet off muddy paths – considered very old fashioned even then), electric irons, plaster of Paris, sputum wire trays, tea urn on stand, cutlery, sterilising bags, medicine cups, fire escape ladders, household refrigerators, sewing machine, vacuum cleaner, door mats, a seat weighing machine, laundry hampers, letter racks, office sundries, china inhalers, surgical requisites, dressing cases, forceps, lino, fire hose, pulley blocks, tools and timber.[9] Dr Wells established a steady routine at Craig-y-nos but in 1926 he fell ill and was replaced the following year by Dr Lizzie Robertson Clark and her Assistant Medical Officer, Dr Sarah Walker. Both doctors were Scottish and had trained at Edinburgh University.

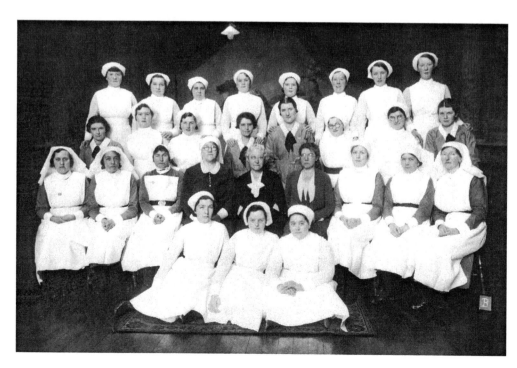

Craig-y-nos staff, mid-1930s. Dr Lizzie Clark (centre) is flanked by the matron (left) and Assistant Medical Officer, Dr Sarah Walker. The woman immediately behind the two doctors is Amy Evans, a teacher, then in her early twenties. She died of TB in 1943. Courtesy Moira Paterson.

TB I've got.

You know what TB signifies?

Totally buggered. He laughed.

His sister cried.

Dannie Abse

Children's stories

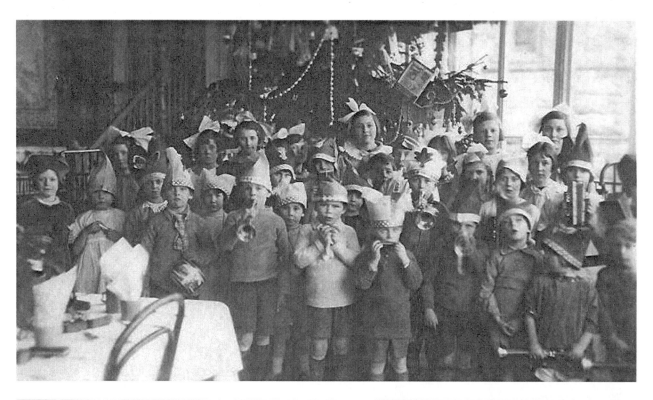

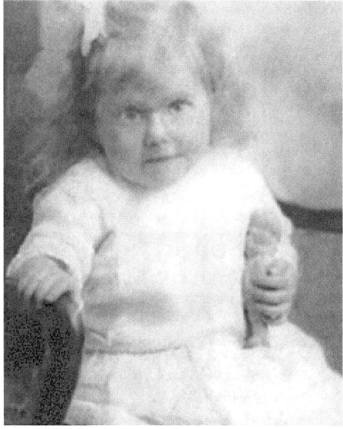

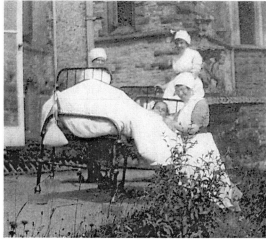

Christmas party in the Glass
Conservatory, 1928. Thomas
is the fourth child from left.
Courtesy Thomas Edward Isaac.

Winnie in Craig-y-nos, aged two.
Courtesy Winnie Gardiner.

Child in bed outside the Glass
Conservatory, c.1924. The foot of the
bed is raised on brick blocks and the
weighted sandbag keeps the child's leg
elevated. The kneeling nurse is Sister
Margaret Phillips. Courtesy Phil Lewis.

Thomas Edward Isaac – Blowing my trumpet

I went in as a nine-year-old in 1928. My bed was in the Glass Conservatory. There's a photograph of me taken at Christmas time. I'm in the front row, of course. I always tell everybody, 'That's me there blowing my trumpet.'

I was the youngest of seven children. My father died in the Spanish 'flu epidemic (1918). We were living in Pontycymer, in the Garw Valley – nothing but mines. It wasn't easy to travel about and my visitors didn't come very often. Of course, they brought sweets but no child was allowed to keep their sweets and chocolates. They were all put into a container and the staff would share them out every so often. There was a lake, which I could see from the windows, and the nurses had a punt - a little boat - and they used to go there in their off-duty time. One of the doctors had a car, and one day he was going to Swansea on business and took a little girl and me on the dickie seat in the back, out in the open, and we had ice cream.

I was looked after good but there was no treatment in Craig-y-nos. You were in bed or just walking around the theatre. You weren't doing any exercises. There were no teachers. Later, I was sent to Talgarth (the South Wales Sanatorium) for a few years where you were put on a certain job, like working on the hospital allotment for the week, and then you were weighed and examined all over. You could also join the Cubs and Boy Scouts but there was nothing like that in Craig-y-nos. When I left school at fourteen, I was supposed to work in the colliery – it was the hungry thirties – but I joined the rest of my family farming at Llwynhendy, near Llanelli, where my mother was born. I didn't get any pay for a year, just my keep, and they bought clothes for me, which wasn't very often. Later, when I was called up to join the army, I discovered I had never had TB after all! I think some children in the early days at Craig-y-nos had other things apart from tuberculosis, such as asthma.

I married a farmer's daughter in 1940 and went into the mines during the war. Eventually, I had the chance of a job with the National Coal Board and ended up a deputy manager of the Mines Rescue Station. My wife died fifteen years ago but I've got a son and daughter, and five grandchildren.

Winnie Gardiner (Gammon) – Growing up in Craig-y-nos

I was admitted at nine months of age in 1927, so I grew up in Craig-y-nos, in the Glass Conservatory. My mother used to visit me twice a year, not that I knew her anyway. The family was 'on the parish' and that is all they were allowed. They thought I had TB of the stomach. Of course, I spent so much time in bed, I ended up being very delicate with such skinny legs - walking around in calipers.

The nurses seemed very old to me and they wore heavy clothing - navy blue or black frocks. If you were naughty and giggling when everybody was supposed to be going to sleep, they'd say, 'Right, any more of this nonsense and out on the veranda you go.' I was always on the veranda. We would stay there all night with a bit of tarpaulin over the cot. In the morning they would take us in to get dressed. I can't remember what clothes I wore but we did change into a frock or a skirt or something. They'd wash us and give us breakfast. The food was horrible. The smell was all over the place. It smelled like lamb stew! But that's what we learned to live on.

There was no schooling. I can't remember drawing or writing on paper. I don't remember ever seeing a book. I don't remember having a doll or a teddy bear, except the big one on the wall brought in by the local mayor one Christmas. We were very restricted - no shouting and no running up and down the ward. Sometimes, nurses would come and sit by children who were crying or hurting. We stayed in until they opened the doors and told us we could go out for half an hour or an hour depending on the weather. Oh, we loved it. We went mad! I can't remember being miserable. I just thought it was home. I never knew about school, or buses, or trains, or my mother, or the village where we lived, Limeslade. I had no thought of the outside world, unlike the older girls. My mother told me that she would cry every time she got to Craig-y-nos because she couldn't come back for six months or a year. The biggest shock was coming home, sitting outside the bungalow and wondering who my four brothers were. After I started school I found out what an orphanage was and I thought, 'Well, they're very much like we were in hospital.' They came in at a certain time, they went out at a certain time, they had food at a certain time, and they went to bed at a certain time, which is not what happens in a home.

I never told anyone that I'd had TB because I wanted to go into the RAF. I was in the RAF from 1944 until 1947 and I enjoyed every minute of it. I married in December 1947 and I've got four children. Grandchildren? Dozens! For most of my life if I changed my diet in any way - had something richer or something I wasn't used to - I would always have a bad stomach. Twenty years ago, I was diagnosed with coeliac disease and needed only to be on a gluten free diet. Instead, I spent the first five years of my life in a TB sanatorium.

Nan Davies - Patti 'ghost' helps child singer

Eleven-year-old Nan Davies was in Craig-y-nos during the winter of 1928-1929. One day the children were to give a concert to the parents on Visiting Day and a young girl with a good voice was picked to sing a solo. Nan, with the second best voice, was to be her stand-in. When the big day came, the soloist was taken ill and Nan had to take her place. She was very nervous standing in the wings until somebody tapped her on the shoulder and she looked around to see a lady wearing an old dress with a bustle, and her hair in a bun, standing behind her. She told her not to worry - that she was going to sing as she had never sung in her life.

Nan went on stage and gave the best performance of her life. The audience was ecstatic and clapped wildly. Nan rushed backstage to thank the lady but there was nobody there except a nurse. Nan believes it was the ghost of Madame Adelina Patti.

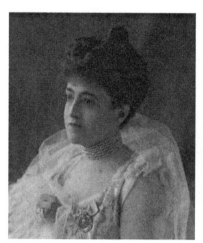

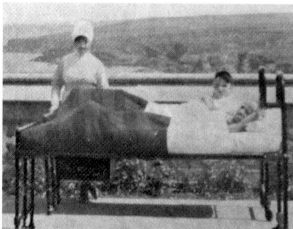

Adelina Patti, 1905.
Adelina Patti A21
© Brecknock Museum
& Art Gallery

Children on the balcony of Kensington Hospital, Pembrokeshire. It was formerly the home of Lord Kensington and given by him to the WNMA. In WNMA booklet, c.1932. Courtesy Llyfrgell Genedlaethol Cymru/ National Library of Wales.

Edward Ellis Thomas - Mice and rats scuttling

At the age of two, in 1923, I was seen to be limping on my right leg. TB hip was diagnosed and I was sent to Kensington Hospital, St Brides Bay, Pembrokeshire. I was strapped to a horizontal frame resting on a four-wheeled wickerwork carriage. There were rumours that my hip ball had dissolved and that an eminent specialist in Liverpool had sent for my X-ray plates out of interest. In 1928, with my parents, I travelled by train from Swansea to Pen-y-cae where we were met by a black ambulance and taken to Craig-y-nos. On my second afternoon we were all carried down to a picnic by the river Tawe. I remember rice pudding with burnt milk-skin and hard boiled eggs.

At certain periods of the year our beds were carried out to the roofed veranda adjoining the ward. Our bed clothes had tarpaulin covers to protect them from the dew. In fine weather, dawn on the veranda was beautiful - fresh, nose-tingling air, all silent apart from awakening farm animals, foxes and birdsong. My parents and others would bring me parcels of comics – *Puck*, *Tiger Tim*. Running beneath the beds were heating pipe ducts with ornamental cast iron covers. We would wet tiny paper pellets in our mouths and drop them through the covers to hear the mice and rats scuttle. My own pinnacle of achievement was playing one of the Seven Dwarfs - on crutches - in the famous Patti theatre. To torment us, the older boys told us we would have our bones scraped, and that at midnight the sculpted figures of fairies, arranged around the ornamental fountain outside, would come to life and dance to eerie music.

I remember George from Pontadawe - he seemed always to be standing on his bed in a long white night-dress with one arm bent at the elbow in a metal frame. Glenys Evans, with dark curly hair like a pretty little doll, was the ward flirt, who 'married' each of us boys in turn. There were three lady doctors. Dr (Lizzie) Clarke, the senior, was an elderly Scot, white-haired with specs and a little Scottie terrier at her heel. Dr (Sarah) Walker was tall with upswept hair. The youngest had Eton-cropped hair and always sat on my bed and made a big fuss of me. I remember Sister Dowey, tall and dark, to whom my parents took a big liking - she came to tea with us at home after my discharge. The hospital engineer, in a yellow boiler-suit, was tall with shiny dark hair neatly swept back. He looked after the generator-engine - the exhaust 'phut-phut-phutting' from the chimney. The engineer always called our heads 'yer knowledge boxes.'

In the early 1960s, suffering with lower back pain, I asked my GP for X-rays of my hip to see if this was a possible cause. The consultant concerned told me that I had never had hip disease but was born with a dislocated hip! I have a shorter right leg, withered and with a stiff knee. This has not prevented me leading a more or less normal life and pursuing a satisfactory and lucrative professional career as a civil engineer with the local government.

Bridie Ronan - A real fairy-tale castle

My back problem recurred in 1927 (at the age of seven) and I was sent to Craig-y-nos. Following a lengthy assessment by Dr (Lizzie) Clark, the Medical Superintendent, and two other doctors, I was carried by a porter to the X-ray department. Next day I had a plaster cast made, which was moulded to the shape of my body, from neck to feet. It was designed to immobilize my lumbar region and legs while allowing limited movement for my arms. It was well padded and fairly comfortable, and I was raised one foot above the mattress on wooden blocks to provide access for the excellent nursing procedures. The beds also had large castors to give easier movement when needed.

Those of us with bone problems lived outside on the balcony in all weathers. Even so, I was thrilled to be in a real fairy-tale castle. Our balcony was home to ten young females, all in plaster beds. On my left was teenager Agnes Jenkins from Abercrave. She had kyphosis (a curvature of the spine). I really pitied her, but Agnes was a strong character and coped well. We all suffered from back pain but my own was very slight compared to others and it wasn't long before I became pain free. Sometimes at night, when I heard my little friends groaning and often screaming, I got upset and cried for them. In fine weather our beds were pushed up to the balcony rails where it was like being in a beautiful enchanted garden. I remember a babbling brook and trees, with bushes and flowering plants. In bad weather each bed was covered with a tarpaulin sheet and we were pushed against the castle walls.

Sometimes, local groups came to entertain us, and the porters would wheel our beds along the corridors to Madame Patti's splendid theatre. When I had regained my mobility I took part in a play in the theatre called 'The Balloon Man', performed by the young patients. I did the prologue. Years later, Betty Maitland-Smith, our next door neighbour in Sketty (Swansea), remembered Adelina Patti as a family friend. She often showed me the lovely china doll she was given as a child by Madame Patti. Mum and Bridge visited every Sunday, making the long journey up the valley by coach. One Sunday they arrived with a huge dolls' house that had all the mod cons, including electric lamps. It filled a large table and we loved playing with it.

I shall never forget the day when Dr Clark told my mum that I had made a remarkable recovery and could come out of plaster. In a week I managed to stand up on my own and after a few sessions of massage, I was well and truly on my feet. Dr Clark said that I could look forward to going home as long as I promised to wear a spinal support.

Bridie worked as a nurse in Swansea before marrying and rearing six children. At the age of seventy-five she climbed Mount Sinai in Egypt.

Right
Boy lying on a plaster bed. The plaster cast can just be seen beneath his left shoulder. His pillow is raised on a block. Courtesy Mari Friend.

Opposite page
Forecourt of Craig-y-nos Castle showing the fountain and goldfish pond, c.1900. In Craig-y-nos Castle estate brochure, 1901. Courtesy Llyfrgell Genedlaethol Cymru/National Library of Wales.

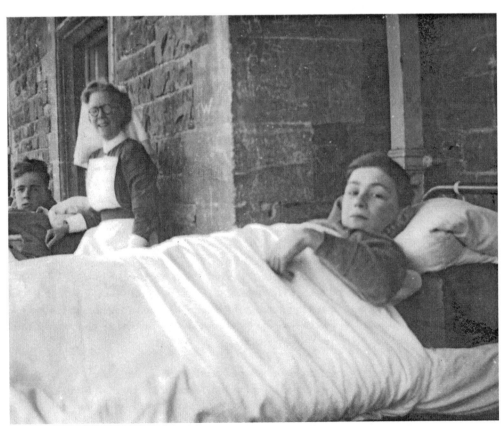

Glynne Lowe - A miserable damn place

I made the long journey from Bronllys via Brecon to Craig-y-nos as a six-year-old in 1927. At Pen-y-cae station an ambulance was waiting to take me to the hospital. I have no memory of treatment, apart from lying in bed, though I do remember having red sores on my legs and I still have the marks today. I don't think my mother came to visit me but cousins from Aberdare did. I have no memories of the food although I recall eating at a table at one end of the ward. They kept sweets there, and we were given sweets after dinner. I don't remember being cold - you don't feel the cold when you're a kid.

Christmas was a highlight. I remember being entertained in the Adelina Patti theatre by Harold Elston, who was a ventriloquist, and Mr Whitney, a butcher who did conjuring tricks. At the end of the performance there was a big box of sweets thrown to the children. We may have had lessons but not many. I remained at Craig-y-nos for seven months. I didn't like it much. It was a miserable damn place. I was transferred to Talgarth (the South Wales Sanatorium) for a further five months where I enjoyed the camaraderie - they were quite a bunch of boys. I sometimes wonder if I really did have TB. I've had pernicious anaemia for forty or fifty years and I think my illness might have been a sign of that.

I started work at fourteen as a motor mechanic but after an accident, which smashed my toes, I sold tractors for a firm run by Harold Elston! In the course of my work I would pass Craig-y-nos and would go into the forecourt to look at the goldfish in the pond. I worked for Elston for fifty years but never once mentioned that I'd seen him performing at Craig-y-nos. Well, you never talked about TB in those days, did you?

Will Davies - Child's comfort from passing train

An old railway man, Dai Hopkins of Cadoxton, remembers the child of another railway man who was in Craig-y-nos in the 1920s.

Whenever a train passed by above the castle, each driver would toot on his whistle. In those quiet days it was easily audible and gave the child so much reassurance that her parents were thinking of her.

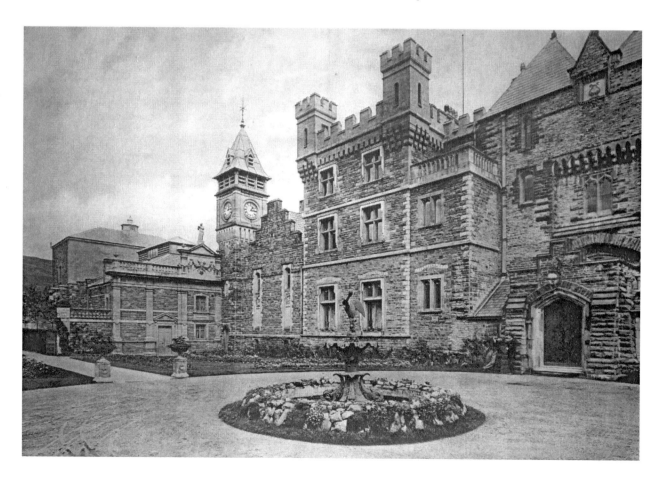

Relatives' stories

Doreen Farley – Tarpaulin bed covers

My sister was a patient in Craig-y-nos and died on 2 March 1924. She would have been eighteen-years-old on 31 March that year. When I visited with my mother (my dad had died of TB in Talgarth – the South Wales Sanatorium - in 1916), there was a young Irish girl in the next bed who was very ill. Her sister used to visit her. I can remember that my mother always took things for the young girl as she did for my sister.

My sister's bed was close to double doors which opened out on to a veranda where there were beds out in the open with tarpaulin on top of the bed clothes. For an eight-year-old like me, I couldn't understand it. I thought it was terrible. Of course, in later years, I learnt all the reasons.

Bridget Robson – Mother's sixth birthday

My mother, Moira Grace Morgan, of Garden City, Llangennech, was in Craig-y-nos in 1924. She was suffering from acute asthma at the time and was sent there for the 'clean fresh air'. However, it was not to be one of her favourable memories. I do not think they were that kind in those days. She was born on 23 December 1918 and spent her sixth birthday there. The Christmas tree in the photograph is decorated with all the toys that the parents and visitors brought in and handed over to staff to put under the tree. My mother says she never got the doll her mother brought in - so sad.

Bridget Robson lives in Northumberland.

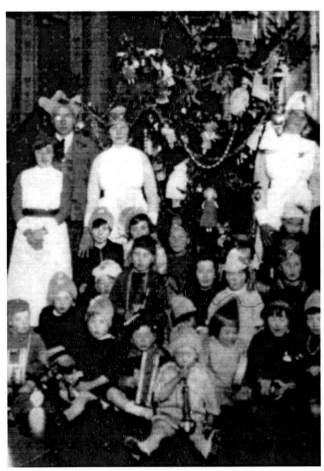

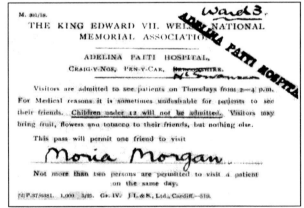

Left
Moira Morgan is seated second left, third row, wearing a white hat with a tassel. Courtesy Bridget Robson.

Moira Morgan's visitor pass. In the 1920s, visiting was once a week for two hours and visitors were allowed to bring tobacco to their friends. The association between smoking and lung disease was not a public health issue until the1950s. Courtesy Bridget Robson.

Opposite page
Craig-y-nos c.1900, by which time Patti had greatly extended the estate to include a fabulous winter garden with exotic flowers and birds (bottom right). In Craig-y-nos Castle estate brochure, 1901. Courtesy Llyfrgell Genedlaethol Cymru/ National Library of Wales.

Sister Margaret Phillips with a young patient, c.1922. Courtesy Phil Lewis.

Staff stories

Phil Lewis - Sister Margaret Phillips and the new hospital

The haunting sound of hymns resonating across the Swansea Valley, sung by patients on the balconies of Craig-y-nos Castle, is one of my earliest memories. I would stand on a rock and listen on Sunday evenings in my home village of Penwyllt, high up the mountain above the castle. My mother, Sister Margaret Phillips, was one of the first members of staff. She was responsible, along with the first matron, for helping convert the former home of Adelina Patti into a TB sanatorium.

My mother had wanted to be a professional musician and she was an accomplished pianist. Instead, she trained as a nurse at Merthyr Tydfil and then did private and military nursing on the south coast during the First World War. When they were opening Craig-y-nos, somebody suggested that she apply for the job because she came from South Wales. She remained at Craig-y-nos from 1921 to 1924, and then gave it up to have her children. She returned in the mid-1930s to work part-time. She used to walk down the mountain from Penwyllt to the castle, even in the depths of winter, taking the short cut through the Patti grounds and over the bridge, a distance of a mile and a quarter over rough terrain. After her nursing shift, she made the return journey up the mountain. Mother was well known for her charity work, and during the Second World War she organized regular concerts and choirs (ex-patients and staff recall Sister Phillips giving piano recitals at the castle)

Craig-y-nos, built in 1842, was originally a private house before Patti took it over. In fact, my oldest school friend, who lives in Cardiff, says that it was part of his family at one time. It didn't have the clock tower or anything then although it was a big, posh house for South Wales. Patti added the Winter Garden (since moved to Swansea and known as the Patti Pavilion). It was at the back of the hospital and it was like Kew Gardens, full of exotic plants. When Patti was there, my father was a boy living up in Penwyllt. She used to have big dinner parties with all sorts of musical stars from Europe staying in the castle, and on big musical weekends she'd encourage the boys from the village to go down with jugs because she knew there'd be far too much soup. They used to walk home with jugs of spare soup. There were lots of pretty maids in the castle! I remember hearing stories - whether true or not - that Adelina Patti's chef used to chase the local lads away with a carving knife. When Patti died, all the lads were heartbroken until it re-opened as a hospital. Suddenly, it was full of pretty nurses, and my father married one!

Sister Margaret Phillips was appointed to Craig-y-Nos on 1 July 1921 at a salary of £62 10 shillings a year, increased to £70 on 1 April 1922. She died in Craig-y-nos in 1985, aged ninety-two. By this time it had become a hospital for the elderly.

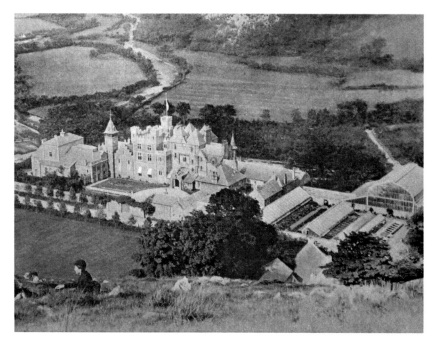

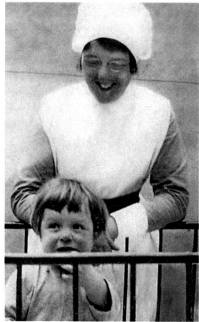

When Patti died, all the lads were heartbroken until it re-opened as a hospital. Suddenly, it was full of pretty nurses, and my father married one!

Phil Lewis

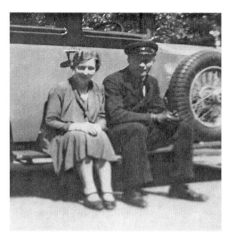

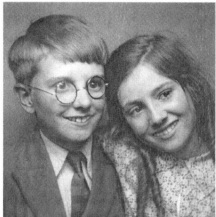

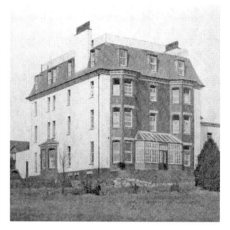

1930s

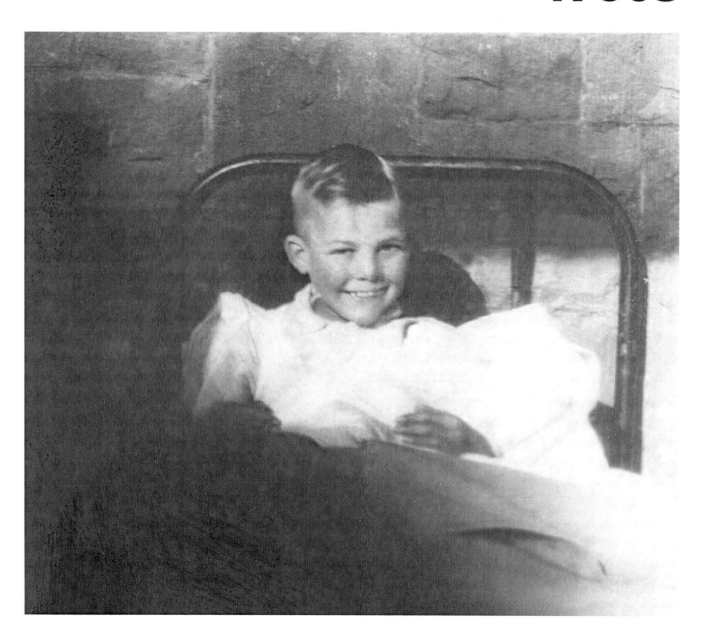

Instant sunshine – Craig-y-nos, TB and treatment in the 1930s

By 1930, there were thirty-eight resident staff at Craig-y-nos and 104 beds.[1] However, waiting lists for sanatorium beds in Wales were high – between 300 and 350 – which put pressure on institutions to increase bed capacity. Craig-y-nos squeezed another twenty-two beds into accommodation intended for staff, some of whom were re-housed in refurbished estate cottages. Four ward blocks accommodated thirty-three men and boys, sixty-three women and girls, and thirty infants.[2] A further fifty beds could be installed by overcrowding, and the hospital was always full.[3] Dr Lizzie Clark, the Medical Superintendent, had two assistant medical officers, Dr Sarah Walker and Dr Maurice Quinlan. Visiting consultants in other specialties were available as required, and the dentist, Mr Jenkyn Evans, who had a private practice in Ystalyfera, held a clinic at Craig-y-nos once a month. Until 1934, an old greenhouse served as the plaster room and light therapy department. Light therapy, or artificial sunshine, was considered beneficial in the treatment of tuberculosis of the skin, glands and bones. A Danish physician, Niels Ryberg Finsen, had developed this form of therapy in Denmark in the 1890s, using powerful carbon arc lamps, and won a Nobel Prize for his work in 1903. The light room at Craig-y-nos was fitted with carbon arc, mercury vapour and Kromeyer (water-cooled ultraviolet radiation) lamps. As well as providing a morale-boosting shot of instant sunshine, these lamps emitted strong ultra-violet rays, and ultra-violet light was known to kill the tuberculosis bacteria. Children with TB of the bones and joints often had their affected limbs immobilised in splints or plaster casts. It was believed that resting the parts would promote healing. Immobilisation on plaster beds for people with TB of the lungs seems to have been developed at Craig-y-nos. This was referred to as 'absolute rest treatment' and entailed lying on a cast moulded to the body for three months or more, wearing minimal garments for hygiene purposes. It was meant to ease symptoms and help damaged lung tissues to heal. Massage to keep the skin and muscles healthy was part of the routine.[4]

Another form of treatment popular at this time was collapse therapy or artificial pneumothorax (AP). This was based on the idea that by collapsing and resting the lung, the TB lesions would have more chance of healing. The technique was developed by an Italian doctor, Carlo Forlanini, in 1882, and introduced into Britain in 1910 by Claude Lillingston, a doctor who had caught TB and been treated by the procedure in Norway. It involved injecting air through a hollow needle into the pleural cavity, which is the gap between the lung and the chest wall. Once the cavity was filled with air, the lung, being spongy and elastic, collapsed down and stopped working. However, because it naturally inflated after a while, the procedure needed to be repeated at intervals ranging from a week to several months. These were called 'refills'. Although collapse therapy had become routine by the 1930s, it was not without dangers. The injection of air into a lung by mistake (causing an air embolism) could have serious, even fatal consequences. Sometimes a lung was partially collapsed permanently in an operation called 'phrenic avulsion'. The phrenic nerve runs through the diaphragm, which is the large muscle beneath the lungs that rises up and down when breathing. Removal of a small section of the phrenic nerve on the right or left side paralyses that half of the diaphragm and partially collapses the lung. This is the operation that Ann Shaw had before being put to lie on her side for a whole year. At Craig-y-nos, there were X-ray facilities for visualising the success or failure of AP, and many procedures were performed on out-patients because the sanatorium had the central after-care clinic for the Brecon and Radnor areas. Nevertheless, the enthusiasm for collapse therapy was not always matched by its success rate. Dr Clark remarked in 1935, that when pneumothorax was undertaken, it was on the assumption that patients had nothing to lose but everything to gain.[5] In other words, it was better to be seen to be doing something than nothing.

Previous page

The chauffeur and his wife who sent Horace books in Craig-y-nos, perhaps along with this photograph. Since he did not receive the books, it is unlikely that he saw the photo. Courtesy Powys Archives.

Gwanwyn and her brother, at about the time she was admitted to Craig-y-nos, 1931. Courtesy, Gwanwyn Evans.

The private hotel known as 'Highland Moors', Llandrindod Wells, was purchased by the Welsh National Memorial Association in 1931 as a rehabilitation centre for sixty boys. In WNMA booklet, c.1932. Courtesy Llyfrgell Genedlaethol/ National Library of Wales.

Haydn, aged seven, in his bed on the balcony of Ward 1, 1931. Courtesy Haydn Beynon.

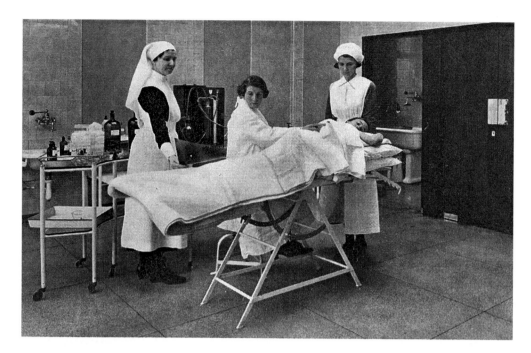

Child having artificial pneumothorax (collapsed lung) in an operating theatre at Stannington Sanatorium, Northumberland, 1930s. Wellcome Images, London.

Many people who were children in Craig-y-nos recall with loathing the procedure known as 'gastric lavage'. The accounts by Roy Harry and Jeanette Evans make harrowing reading, and many have asked why this was done. The technique seems to have originated in the children's department at the Hôpital Hérold, Paris, in the early 1930s, and was used to search for tuberculosis bacteria in children with pulmonary (lung) infection. Most children cannot expectorate (cough up phlegm) from the lungs. Instead, they swallow it so that it ends up in the stomach. This can be retrieved by washing out the stomach with warm water poured through a funnel on the end of a rubber tube pushed down the throat. Once the stomach juices had been captured they were usually injected into specially bred guinea-pigs, which reacted positively or negatively depending on the presence or absence of TB germs. TB germs in sputum indicated active disease and the child would be infectious. The French doctors claimed that the procedure caused little inconvenience to children but, for the most part, the oral testimonies in this book reveal otherwise.[6] Nevertheless, it was considered important to keep those with TB germs separate from those without (although this was not always the case in Craig-y-nos) and the former did not receive lessons. There were two teachers at Craig-y-nos, Miss Jones, who taught the infants, and Miss Evans, who took the senior class. Amy Evans was appointed to the staff in 1934 at the age of twenty. She was a local girl from Ystradgynlais but lived in the hospital.[7] Unfortunately, she caught tuberculosis and died in 1943.[8]

By the mid-1930s it cost about £23,000 a year to maintain the beds at Craig-y-nos but the building was considered unfit for purpose as a hospital and grossly outdated in terms of basic amenities. A lift serving all floors was installed in 1934 but the main high pressure steam boiler was sixty-years-old, pre-dating Patti's era, and had been considered dangerous years before by His Majesty's Office of Works. There was, in effect, no central heating system at all. The kitchen was similarly antiquated. The Welsh National Memorial Association (WNMA) proposed to abandon Craig-y-nos if the anticipated new hospital in Swansea (Singleton) was ever built, and questioned the wisdom of spending money on it in the meantime.[9] Although the site at Singleton had been acquired by the WNMA in 1912, delay in construction of a purpose-built TB hospital was not due entirely to financial constraints in this decade of economic depression. Swansea residents objected to the threat of tuberculosis on their doorsteps. In 1935 they protested to the Ministry of Health, and the Vicar of Sketty called it a 'suicidal policy'.[10] Better by far to keep patients isolated in the upper reaches of the Tawe valley, twenty-three miles from the city. The Craig-y-nos House Committee (undoubtedly aware of local politics), which oversaw the daily running of the sanatorium and made recommendations for improving the comfort of patients and staff, pushed for certain works to be prioritised. Eventually, in 1937, the WNMA agreed to spend £15,000 over the following five-year period on centralising the boiler plant, replacing a children's ward, converting a staff bungalow into a ward block, modernising the kitchen, renewing electrical batteries (the sanatorium was not linked to the national grid), and constructing self-contained quarters suitable for a Medical Superintendent. Dr Lizzie Clarke lived in a two-storey flat within the castle, which was considered unsuitable as a family home and therefore restricted the Association's choice of Superintendent.[11] In fact, Dr Clark retired in October 1937 and her assistant, Dr Sarah Walker, left with her. The new Medical Superintendent was Dr Ivor Williams, whose previous post had been at Glan Ely Hospital, Cardiff. He arrived with his wife, Lyn, but was in post less than two years before being transferred, very reluctantly, to Kensington Hospital, St Brides Bay, Pembrokeshire, an institution for children with non-pulmonary tuberculosis. His transfer came about because the Medical Superintendent of North Wales Sanatorium, Dr David Fenwick Jones, was unwell and had been advised to 'ease down'.

As he had given long and loyal service to the WNMA, it was thought appropriate to cushion his last years, without loss of status, in a post considered to be less stressful.[12] Dr Fenwick Jones remained at Craig-y-nos until his retirement in 1947, when Dr Williams returned with his wife and two young daughters, also becoming Tuberculosis Officer for the area.

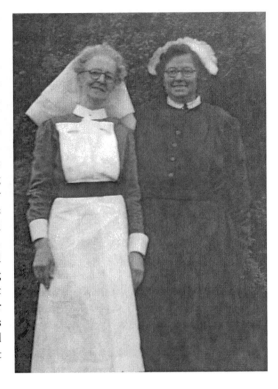

A number of staff employed in sanatoria, at least those in direct contact with patients, had themselves recovered from tuberculosis. One who would have been known to Fenwick Jones was Ethel Outram, appointed as a staff nurse to North Wales Sanatorium in 1921, who then spent a number of years on and off as a patient. She was transferred to Craig-y-nos in 1930 and remembered as strict and fearsome, but she nevertheless would have appreciated her patients' needs and difficulties.[13] Because many of the nurses who came to Craig-y-nos had trained in sanatoria they were not State Registered. State registration had been established in 1919 and the examinations for entry to the Register were administered by the General Nursing Council, which did not recognise training in tuberculosis nursing. By the 1930s, nurses in sanatoria could train for the two-part Tuberculosis Association examination. Part I consisted of anatomy, physiology and hygiene, and part II was concerned with nursing and tuberculosis. Sister Mary Knox Thomas, who later became Matron, was appointed as Sister Tutor in 1936 and therefore largely responsible for training probationer nurses for these exams.[14] Nurses such as Valerie Brent (Price), who wished to become State Registered, had to leave for general nursing training in an approved hospital. Turberculosis nurses were not necessarily any less dedicated than their colleagues in general nursing but their jobs carried less prestige in the nursing world and it was often difficult to recruit girls who wanted to be career nurses.

Death rates from tuberculosis in England and Scotland dropped sharply between 1900 and 1935. In Scotland, for example, whereas twenty-two people out of every 10,000 died of TB in 1900, the numbers were seven by 1935. In England, the numbers dropped from seventeen to seven, but in Wales, they dropped from eighteen to nine.[15] To epidemiologists (people who study diseases in whole populations), these figures were worrying because they indicated that Wales was lagging behind the rest of Britain in controlling tuberculosis. Indeed, the Welsh counties of Glamorgan, Radnor, Pembroke, Montgomery, Anglesey, Cardigan, Brecon, Merioneth and Carnarfon had the highest TB death rates in the whole of Wales and England, apart from London.[16] The situation was not helped by the attitudes of influential doctors such as Professor S Lyle Cummins, the WNMA's Director of Research at the Welsh National School of Medicine, who went on to become the David Davies Professor of Tuberculosis. He blamed the characteristics of the Welsh – their close family relationships, customs and social habits (such as addiction to tea and overeating on Sundays) and their fatalistic outlook.[17] In reality, areas with high tuberculosis rates, and rates that were not falling as rapidly as national rates, generally coincided with those most adversely affected by unemployment and economic depression. Furthermore, TB killed the young productive members of society, most particularly the age group fifteen to twenty-five. In 1939, out of every 100 deaths in this age group in Wales, thirty-one men and fifty-three women died from TB.[18] Many ex-patients from the 1920s and 30s recall rumours that admission to Craig-y-nos was a certain death sentence – if you had 'the consumption you went to Craig-y-nos to die.' Since so few records relating to the hospital have survived, it is not possible to discover accurate death rates except for the year 1934, in which fifteen per cent of patients died. Of these, 12.5 per cent were adults, and the ratio of adults to children that year was exactly 50:50.[19] Death rates from tuberculosis in children up to the age of fourteen were never as high as they were in adults.

Vernon Evans and Peter Wagstaffe recall that patients' diets were augmented by game and fish caught on the Craig-y-nos estate. There was also a very large kitchen garden and greenhouses growing fruit and vegetables for the sanatorium, and hens were kept for eggs. Some food items were bulk purchased by the WNMA for use throughout its organisation, which by 1938 included eighteen hospitals and sanatoria, 100 dispensaries and clinics, a research laboratory, educational centre and central administration. WNMA staff were allowed to purchase items from the central stock at cost price. Whether the WNMA ordered sufficient foodstuffs to meet a staff as well as a hospital demand is unclear but certainly the Marmite Food Extract Company, in 1938, believed that catering tins of Marmite, supplied for the benefit of patients, were being misappropriated into private homes. There was strong and rather arrogant denial from the WNMA, which stated that staff had a right to be so supplied, for their personal use.[20] With a war looming, the temptation to stockpile household rations must have been irresistible.

Children's Stories

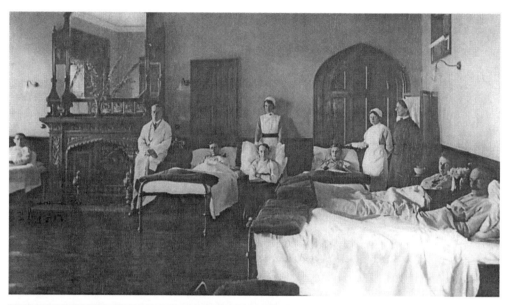

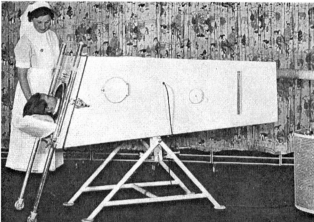

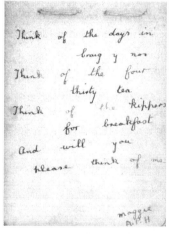

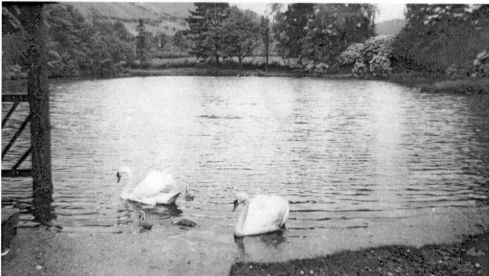

Gwanwyn Evans - Sun-ray treatment, calico pants, and songs

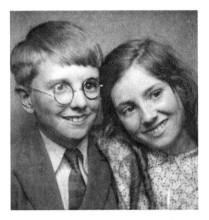

At the age of ten, in November 1931, I developed an abscess on my right jaw, which was identified as tubercular and necessitated my admission to Craig-y-nos. My home was at Builth Wells (Powys). There was no public transport and so the local vicar conveyed me, accompanied by my father, to the hospital. I had to undergo an operation to scrape my jawbone. Treatment necessitated my having a sun-ray lamp applied to the scar. The first application frightened me because a black, strange smelling sheet of something like cardboard was placed on my face. It contained an aperture for my scar but the rest had to protect my face against the sun-ray. Each morning I had the scab 'torn away', the bleeding stopped with methylated spirits - did that smart? - and the heat applied. I was in hospital for sixteen weeks and this continued for that period of time. All the children, boys and girls, went each morning to the Sun-ray Room, wearing only little calico pants and goggles and we sat around, had games or sang songs around the big sun-ray lamp.

Christmas was approaching and we were rehearsed for a musical playlet. I had a very good singing voice and consequently had the lead. My mother posted my best frock, a pretty pink knitted silk with flared skirt. Sadly, though, on the morning of the event, I was found to have a temperature and had to remain in bed while another girl took my place! As a consolation I was taken around the other wards to sing. My party piece in those days was 'When it's spring time in the Rockies'. Lord David Davies of Llandinam (David Davies, MP, later Lord Davies of Llandinam, was the first president of the Welsh National Memorial Association) came to the hospital as Father Christmas. We had in our 'stockings' a tin of toffees and a tablet of soap. My present from Father Christmas was a doll, which I kept for ten years. Christmas afternoon we were taken to the babies' ward - Adelina Patti's Glass Conservatory - where a large Christmas cracker suspended from the ceiling was lowered and we all lined up at each end to give an enormous pull, from which poured presents. I had a set of doll's furniture.

In 1981/82 Gwanwyn Evans became the first lady mayoress of the Borough of Brecknock. She lives in Aberyscir, near Brecon.

Squash, squash, squash!

'If you were reprimanded in Craig-y-nos it was called "squash",' says Gwanwyn Evans. 'One girl, Madge, wrote a poem which we used to sing when out of hearing of the staff!'

Squash, squash, squash, here comes Staff Nurse to squash us.
Squash, squash, squash, that's all we're getting here
The nurses and the sisters,
Their tongues must be in blisters.
That's all we get in Craig-y-nos is
Squash, squash, squash!

Many years later my husband saw Madge in Brecon. She had become a Sergeant in the ATS and was marching her recruits around the town. It was obvious that her stay in Craig-y-nos had been beneficial!

Gwanwyn and her brother, at about the time she was admitted to Craig-y-nos, 1931. Courtesy, Gwanwyn Evans.

Pages from Margaret Ritchie's autograph book, *c.*1930 Verses written in autograph books became part of the 'folk lore' of Craig-y-nos and were passed down through the decades. Courtesy Ann Williams.

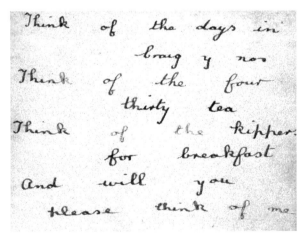

Think of the days in Craig y nos
Think of the four thirty tea
Think of the kipper for breakfast
and will you please think of me.

Oh I love the Swansea Girls
Cause they have teeth like oster pearls
And every time I kiss their ruby lips
They make me smell of fish and chips

Squash, squash, squash!

Squash, squash, squash, here
comes Staff Nurse to squash us.

Squash, squash, squash,
that's all we're getting here

The nurses and the sisters,
Their tongues must be in blisters.

That's all we get in Craig-y-nos
is Squash, squash, squash!

Vernon Evans - Shooting parties and rabbit stew

I was born in 1919, the tenth of fourteen children. I lacked nothing due to the kindness of relatives and friends, but in the early 1930s, just into my teens, I was admitted to Craig-y-nos. At that time, the gentry and the doctors had their shooting parties on a Tuesday, and we the patients lived on rabbit meat and stews for a few days. The food wasn't too bad, until I found a slug on my Brussels sprouts, which put me off them for life.

A lot of people don't understand what we went through. They think we are exaggerating the treatment we received. I was turned down for the war because they told me they didn't want lame ducks in the fighting forces.

Vernon joined the family bakery business, becoming a master baker, and served fifty-three years before retiring. He became a lecturer in Bakery and Confectionery at Bridgend College and for years wrote a weekly column in the *Glamorgan Gazette* about life in the Llynfi Valley.

Extract from letter written to Edward Ellis Thomas. Vernon died seven years ago

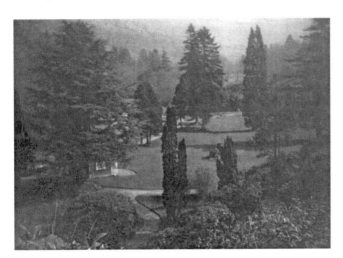 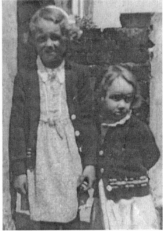

The Craig-y-nos estate comprised forty-eight acres of parkland and woods habouring pheasants, partridges, snipe, duck and other wing and ground game. Courtesy Dulcie Oltersdorf.

Peggy (right) with her sister Betty, before her admission to Craig-y-nos. Courtesy Peggy Tizzard.

Peggy Tizzard (Jones) - Punished if you broke the rules

I was told I was going on holiday and wore a red coat and a red beret. Then they left me in a cot in this big ward with lots of other children. It was 1939 and I was three-years-old. We were not allowed toys so my teacher sent in a slate with a piece of chalk and a box of wooden blocks with faces on them. I spent hours playing with that. After a while they put me upstairs in the women's ward. I was the only child there. I never saw another child for years except once when Dr Jarman brought in his son who was the same age and we spent time rolling this thing down the stairs. We didn't know what it was. Eventually, Dr Jarman came back and picked it up. He said it was an orange, and he peeled it and we ate it.

If you broke the rules you would be punished. Once I ran to the lake and sat on the wooden building throwing sticks into the water at the swans and ducks. They had a big search party to find me. I was punished and tied to the bed. I used to follow Sister (Winnie) Morgan around everywhere. My mother visited one Saturday every month. There was a special bus from Swansea to bring visitors up the valley. My father was in Craig-y-nos too. They said there was no hope for him and my mother took him home to die. I was wrapped in a blanket and taken down to see him for the last time. He hugged me and I cried because he was walking away and I wanted to go with him. He gave me a book, which I was not allowed to keep because of infection. So that was the last gift from my father. I never found that book. We had a radio in the ward and the nurse would give a penny to the person who could guess the speaker of the news each night. Nothing was allowed to be brought in except fruit. Once the village, Crofty, collected all their (war ration) coupons to buy me chocolate biscuits. My mother smuggled them in to me and I ate them and was violently sick. I remember going to see 'Tom Thumb' in the Patti theatre, the first film I ever saw. A woman tried to pick me up to give me a cuddle and I screamed. She was from my village and knew my parents. I can remember having injections every morning. Later, I was told that they were gold and sulphur injections.

When I arrived home in 1941 I found it difficult because the house was full of people. They were neighbours but I didn't recognize them and my father wasn't there. I missed that. So I took my teddy bear and went upstairs to bed.

Peggy became a nursery nurse. Later, she went to Trinity College, Carmarthen, and took a diploma in Education from the University of Swansea.

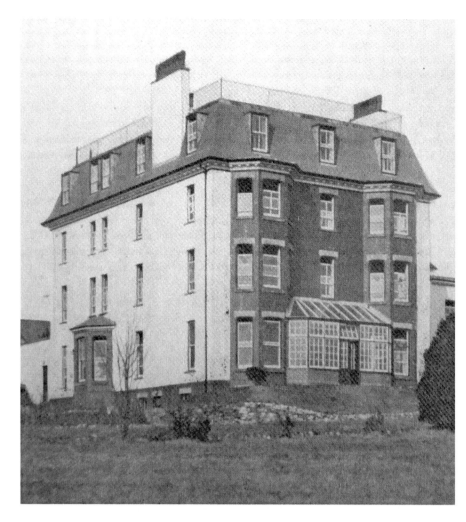

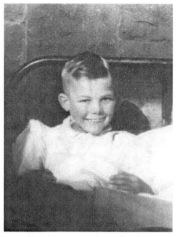

Haydn, aged seven, in his bed on the balcony of Ward 1, 1931. Courtesy Haydn Beynon.

The private hotel known as 'Highland Moors', Llandrindod Wells, was purchased by the Welsh National Memorial Association in 1931 as a rehabilitation centre for sixty boys. In WNMA booklet, *c*.1932. Courtesy Llyfrgell Genedlaethol/National Library of Wales.

Haydn Beynon – Lots of people dying

I saw my parents about every two months. In those days (1931), money was *very* tight. I was one of five children and my father was a collier. It took them three or four hours to travel from Taibach (near Port Talbot) to Craig-y-nos. My bed was on the balcony and I can remember sitting up in bed with pyjamas on and my mother and father with overcoats and scarves and hats on, the snow and the rain coming in, and they'd be shivering. It *was* cold but you didn't feel it after a while. We were allowed out into the grounds. Once, a couple of us children went down towards the edge of the forest, and a fox and hounds came through. It frightened us to death. I have a lifelong hatred of tapioca pudding and semolina as a result of having it in Craig-y-nos. You were given four squares of Cadbury's chocolate, and I didn't qualify because if you didn't eat your afters, you couldn't have chocolate. I can remember vividly … every few days the curtains would go round a bed and porters would wheel somebody away who had died. I was only a youngster but it seemed that there were lots of people dying at that time, like every other day.

Craig-y-nos was monotonous, one day after the other. The difference between Highland Moors, where I went in 1932, and Craig-y-nos is that there you were encouraged to play. I remember playing cricket. It was more like a convalescent home. I missed a lot of schooling. I went down the pit at fourteen. When you look back it's stupid after two years in a sanatorium. I worked underground from fourteen till I was eighteen. One Friday, I came home and said to my mother, 'I've had enough' and I put my working clothes straight on the fire. She helped me burn the whole lot - underwear, shoes, the lot. And my father came in. 'What the bloody hell are you doing?' I had to go down to see the colliery manager. 'Right,' he said, 'You know that you'll be called up for the forces (this would be about 1942).' I said, 'I don't care.' He said, 'Fill this form up with the reasons for leaving.' So I filled it up and said, 'All the water leaking and bad air.' When I took it back, he was out with the pen and whoosh, whoosh, whoosh (deleted all the comments). He said, 'There's no bad air in our colliery.' Within about a fortnight I was called up. I went in the Navy. Marvellous! I enjoyed it. I stayed on after the war ended.

After leaving the navy, Haydn worked in the Port Talbot steel works for over thirty years. He married in 1949 and has two children. His wife died in 2005.

Valerie Williams (Llewellyn) - The broken monkey

Whatever happened to Bridie O'Sullivan, the Irish child abandoned in Craig-y-nos? Valerie's parents had thought of adopting four-year-old Bridie as company for their daughter because they were the same age - until the 'monkey incident'.

Valerie: I had an uncle who worked as a sailor and he brought me back this big wooden toy monkey. But we were not allowed to play with toys because of the fear of infection so they put it at the end of the ward so that everybody could enjoy it and nobody would be jealous. Well, Bridie got out of bed in the night and broke my monkey. I was so angry with her. My parents wanted to adopt her but I wouldn't let them. Bridie had been left in Craig-y-nos by her parents in the mid-thirties when she was about twelve months old.

I have no memory of walking about during my two years there. I remember the big iron cots and looking out through the bars. They would wheel our cots outside. If it started to rain there was a rush to bring them back in. My uncle, who was a bus driver, used to sneak in to visit me when he was passing once a week, and on one occasion he helped to pull the beds back into the Glass Conservatory. We were not allowed to get damp! When I went home in 1940 there was a family celebration. We had a party and when it was over I put on my hat and coat to go back to Craig-y-nos. My mother said to me, 'You are home.' She was upset.

Valerie married and worked as a telephonist in Swansea. She leads an active life swimming, ballroom dancing and going to jazz festivals. But she often wonders what happened to Bridie O'Sullivan.

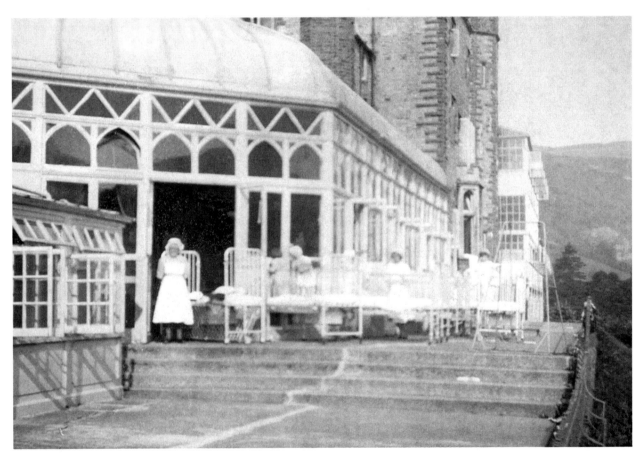

Exterior of the Glass Conservatory with the babies' cots on the terrace. In the background are the balconies with glassed-in side windows. In the foreground (left) are the open windows of the Annexe, the ward for young women. Courtesy Peggy Jones.

Haydn Harris - Iron lungs

My father was married twice. His first wife died of TB at twenty-eight years of age, leaving him with two children. My elder sister had TB when she was twelve years of age and she was in another sanatorium. My cousin living next door died of TB meningitis. I was admitted to Craig-y-nos as a four-year-old in 1937. I was in an all male ward but it was not all children. It had two areas. One was raised. That's where the iron lungs were. I think there were about half a dozen. They were big, at least six foot in length. The only part of the person you could see was the head. It was like a box with a man's head on it. These machines helped 'extreme' patients to breath. Very few patients came down from the platform alive. My bed was down by the window, overlooking the gardens and river. It was lovely sitting on the balcony when the sun was shining. I never felt ill.

There were times during the day you had to rest but we often went out for walks in the grounds. We also used to go walking with the nurses and they would take us down to visit the gardeners' hut where the men used to catch squirrels and keep them in cages so that we could see them. The one person that sticks in my mind is the odd job man on the ward. He was strict but he wouldn't play down to a child. I liked him. In the winter of 1937, a very snowy winter, he was up a ladder doing something just outside my bed and he fell off and injured his arm. He ended up in the next bed to me, just for the night.

It was difficult for my parents to travel from Clyne up the Neath and Swansea Valleys in those days. I was worried when my mother failed to turn up for a couple of months. I began to wonder what had happened to her but when I got home I found I had a baby brother, a few weeks old. After I came out my mother always referred to the fact that I was in hospital 'under observation' though I don't think that was the case. I was one of the first in my village to pass the eleven-plus and go to grammar school. Most of my working life I was with BP (British Petroleum), first as a lab assistant then as a Transport Superintendent. Throughout my thirty years there I only had five days off.

Haydn is married with two boys and three grandchildren, and is an active member of the Port Talbot Writers Club.

Haydn clearly describes 'iron lung' machines. These were respirators that helped people with polio to breathe after their diaphragm muscles had been paralysed by the polio virus. It has not been possible to verify the existence of iron lungs in Craig-y-nos. In 1938, the *Sunday Chronicle* newspaper disclosed the shortage of these respirators – there were only eighteen in Britain. By the end of that year, Lord Nuffield offered to build them in his motor plant at Cowley, Oxford, and he went on to manufacture 800 at a cost of £97 each.

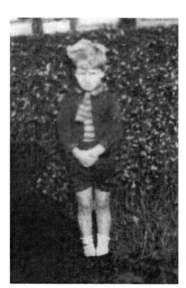

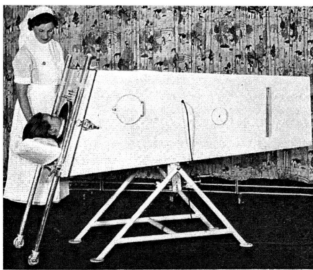

Haydn after his discharge from Craig-y-nos, *c.*1938. Courtesy Haydn Harris.

The Both respirator. This inexpensive machine was manufactured by Lord Nuffield, in his motor plant at Cowley, Oxford, and donated to hospitals in Britain and the Commonwealth. From *Breathing Machines ...* MRC, 1939. Wellcome Images, London.

A lot of people don't understand
what we went through.

They think we are exaggerating
the treatment we received.
I was turned down for the
war because they told me
they didn't want lame ducks
in the fighting forces.

Vernon Evans

Relatives' Stories

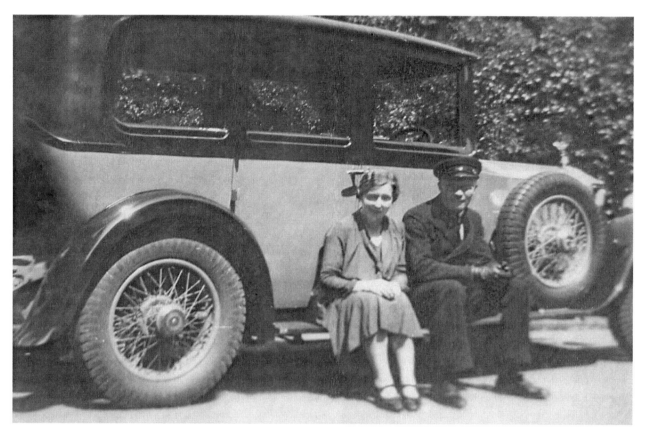

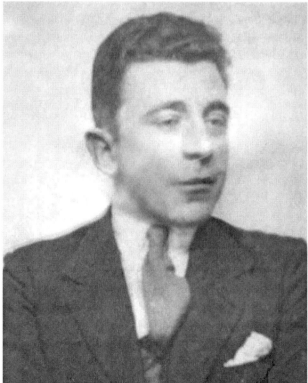

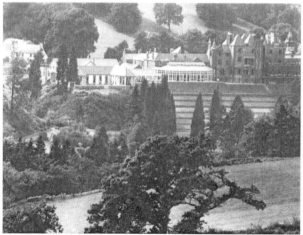

Horace before his admission to Craig-y-nos. Courtesy John Batts and Powys Archives.

The chauffeur and his wife who sent Horace books in Craig-y-nos, perhaps along with this photograph. Since he did not receive the books, it is unlikely that he saw the photo. Courtesy John Batts and Powys Archives.

Train drivers passing Craig-y-nos in the 1930s would have this view of the castle. The railway line was closed in the 1960s. Courtesy Beryl Lewis.

Death certificate from Craig-y-nos, 1930. Courtesy Mabbett.

John Batts – Cousin Horace's last letter

I have some letters written from Craig-y-nos in 1930 by Horace Rees Batts, a cousin of my father, to his family (copies of these letters are in Powys County Archives, Llandrindod Wells). They paint a picture of an oppressive regime for TB patients, typical of that practiced in sanatoria at that time.

'I have been put on absolute rest, which means I must not move in bed, receive no visitors, write no letters, have everything done for me, even to being fed. It is to get my temperature down I suppose. Don't worry, will you?' Horace comments on the weekly 'treat' – listening to the Sunday service on the wireless. 'We had a nice service on wireless Sunday night. I thought of Sunday nights I should have gone to chapel but never did. I wish now I had, but if God will spare me I bet I'll be different. I've said that before, haven't I though?'

Tillie, Horace's sister, who lived in Bournemouth (probably in service), wrote to him regularly. 'Hope you had the parcel safe, and hope you are feeling stronger. I was out yesterday and went to look for the pen, but the shops was closed. You shall have it the first chance I get. I expect you had some books this week and wondered where they came from. It was the chauffeur's wife that sent them. Hope you had them alright.' A subsequent letter from Horace to his sister stated that he was still waiting for the books to arrive. (Some patients, for reasons unknown, never received parcels or letters sent to them, even as late as the 1950s. Gwyn Thomas, a child patient in the early 1940s, found a letter written to him by his mother in his medical file, forty years later).

Horace managed to write another letter without the staff noticing, and persuaded a visitor to post it. 'Dear Mam and all, Just a line on the q.t. Tell Mrs P not to send any more cakes as cakes are not allowed. I shall want some eggs and fruit. You can send bananas, apples etc., but no pears. Sister opens all my letters, parcels, just slits them that's all, so be careful what you are sending. It's a funny business this, being fed and everything. I have gone shiverish but that's to be expected. Remember me to all …' Horace, aged twenty-nine, died soon after this letter was written.

John Batts lives in Australia.

Opposite page

Jacko the peacock displays his plumage. Peacocks had lived on the estate since Adelina Patti's day. Courtesy Mary Watkins.

Caroline 'riding' one of the stone stags on the terrace at the back of the hospital. Courtesy Mari Friend.

Nurse 'Glen' in playful pose. Courtesy Mary Ireland.

Chest X-ray showing severe tuberculosis of the lungs, which are filled with patches of scarred tissue and cavities filled with infectious matter (white areas). The X-ray was taken in the 1930s before there was any effective treatment for TB. Wellcome Images, London.

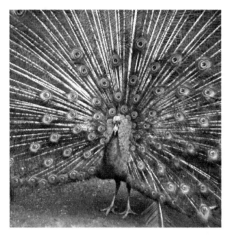
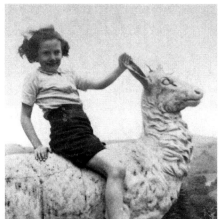
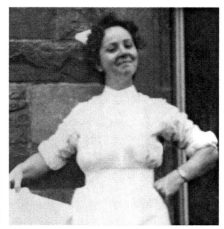

1940s

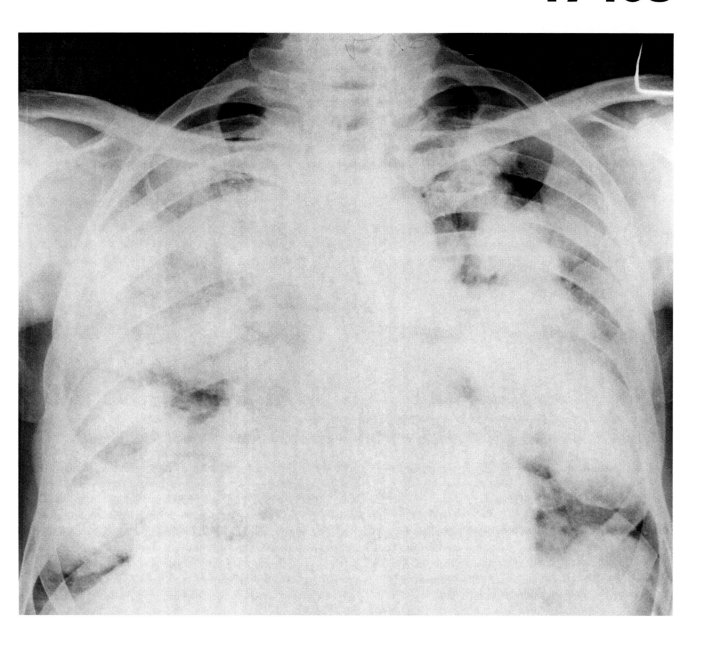

Magic bullets – Craig-y-nos, TB and treatment in the 1940s

By the early 1940s there were 126 beds and seventy-eight staff at Craig-y-nos, of whom about sixty-five were resident. They included three medical staff, thirty-four nurses (all female), twenty-eight domestics, kitchen staff and porters, teaching and clerical staff, engineers, gardeners, a chauffeur, carpenter and painter. The annual wages for the entire staff totalled £7615! Ward maids and student nurses could expect to earn just under £1 a week, sisters about £2.50, and the matron about £4.25. Dr Ivor Williams, who resumed his post as Medical Superintendent in 1947, received an annual salary of just over £1000 after deductions for his residential quarters and garage.[1] Quite separate from the finances required to run the sanatorium, most of which came from the Welsh National Memorial Association (WNMA), was the Patients' Comforts Fund. Money for this was raised or donated by (mostly) local people and organisations which contributed the proceeds of dances, rabbit club shows and whist drives. Collection boxes at working men's clubs, chapels, Sunday schools, secondary schools and collieries were emptied each year into the Fund. A very active fund-raiser was Jenkyn Evans, who had been the dental surgeon at Craig-y-nos since at least the early 1930s (he qualified as a dentist in Bristol in 1922) and also had a private practice in Ystalyfera. In 1944, for example, he was responsible for organising events that raised over £162, nearly forty per cent of the total donations.[2] The Patient's Comforts Fund was supposed to pay for items such as reading material, Christmas gifts and outings, although very few people recall trips beyond the castle walls, and very few are mentioned in the hospital school log book.[3] However, a modern central receiver with headphones was installed in 1948 at a cost of over £1200, of which just under half came from the Fund.[4]

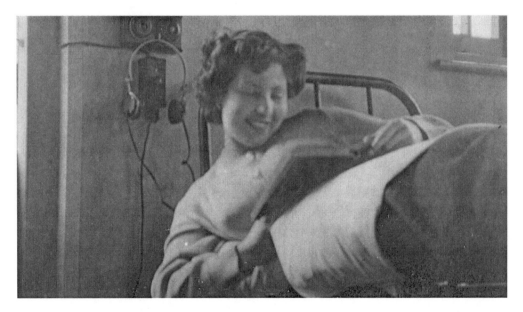

New radio receiver headphones next to her bed although Rachel Davies (Morgan) prefers to read a book. Courtesy Rachel Davies.

The decade witnessed many important changes in the diagnosis and treatment of tuberculosis and of course, in the transfer of services to the Government with the establishment of the National Health Service in 1948. During the war years, 1939-1945, there were increases in the rates of tuberculosis throughout Britain. In Wales, in 1944, there were more than 900 new cases than in 1939.[5] However, in that year, the Welsh National Memorial Association (WNMA) financed a mobile mass radiography unit, which travelled over 2500 miles in its first twelve months and X-rayed some 50,000 people in the search for hitherto undiagnosed cases.[6] A number of children evacuated to the Swansea area from London were admitted to Craig-y-nos and it is likely that they had tuberculosis when they arrived in Wales. Others, like Rose Pugh (Hunt), evacuated locally to an unwelcoming family and underfed, probably caught the infection there. Most of the children in Craig-y-nos had TB of the lungs.[7] In 1945, Matron Knox-Thomas applied to the General Nursing Council (GNC) for Craig-y-nos to be approved as a training school for general nurses who wished to gain experience in children's nursing (the GNC did not recognise training in tuberculosis nursing). This would have raised its status and perhaps made the hospital more appealing to State Registered nurses, the services of whom it seemed impossible to attract. Indeed, the only State Registered nurses at Craig-y-nos were the matron and her deputy. Most of the others had, or were training for, the Tuberculosis Association Certificate (see page 25). Day nurses worked a fifty-four-hour week and night nurses a seventy-two-hour week. Nursing staff had six-monthly chest X-rays and Mantoux tests (skin tests to detect sensitivity to tuberculin) to check that they had not caught tuberculosis. The age of entry for probationer nurses at Craig was eighteen although, in 1945, Valerie Brent (Price) was taken on at the age of fifteen. It is unlikely that the representatives of the GNC who visited the sanatorium in November of that year, would have been aware of this breach in regulations otherwise their report might have been even more critical than it was. There was no attempt, they said, to train nurses properly. In addition, there were no hand washing facilities for them on three of the four ward blocks, apart from the kitchen sink. Neither was any attempt made to sterilise patients' crockery although this was to become less of an infection control issue than nurses' hand washing. The kitchen itself was of a poor standard, as were the patients' sanitary annexes. The key to the drugs cupboard was, apparently, under no one's jurisdiction as it was simply left hanging in the Duty Room. What was most disturbing to the inspectors, however, was the sight of a number of children aged four to eight, and even some younger than this, tied in bed with restrainers. As a consequence of this visit, they did not recommend that Craig-y-nos be granted approval as a training school for nurses.[8]

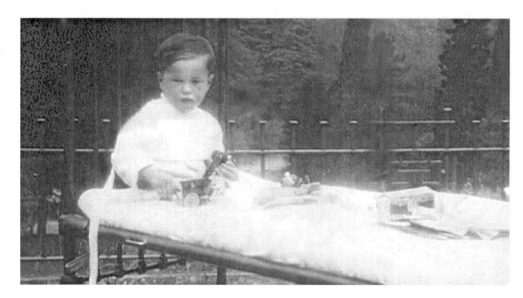

Roger Wyn Beynon is wearing a jacket with restraining ties, which would be fastened to the cot rails to prevent him getting out of bed. Courtesy Roger Wyn Beynon.

An acute shortage of nursing staff by 1946 resulted in the closure of two wards and the transfer of all adult males to the South Wales Sanatorium at Talgarth. In addition, there was only one permanent teacher, Mrs Thomas. School inspectors described her as having an 'impossible task' to teach the three R's (reading, writing and arithmetic), history, geography, nature study, literature, musical appreciation, scripture, arts and crafts to sixty-six pupils aged five to fourteen. Amongst the list of handcrafts were plasticine and cardboard modelling, wood carving, leather and felt work, rug-making, embroidery, knitting, and making Christmas, Easter, Valentine and birthday cards for relatives. Books included *Anderson's* and *Grimm's Fairy Tales*, *The Water Babies* (Charles Kingsley), *Hiawatha* (H W Longfellow), *Alice in Wonderland* (Lewis Carroll), *Children of the New Forest* (Captain Marryat), *King Solomon's Mines* (H Rider Haggard), *Treasure Island* (R L Stevenson), *Lambs' Tales from Shakespeare* and Dickens galore. The inspectors observed that although the stock cupboard was full of books and handicraft materials, there were no facilities for keeping these beside the children's beds, and there were very few toys in evidence. Dr Huppert, the Assistant Medical Officer, was, apparently, very much against bedside lockers because there were not enough staff to keep them tidy. The inspectors were clearly not impressed and considered 'her human approach to the children not always too gentle in manner, especially if the child is unresponsive or fractious.'[9]

Dr Margaret Pauline Huppert (or 'Hubbard' as she was always known to children and staff) came to Craig-y-nos as Assistant Medical Officer in about 1945, from North Wales Sanatorium. Her background is rather mysterious but she was born on 16 August 1893 and qualified as a doctor in Vienna in 1923. She left Austria about the time of the Anschluss, the merger of Austria into Nazi Germany, in 1938. She was on the medical register in Britain in 1942, which was the first year of temporary registration for wartime refugee doctors, and remained at Craig-y-nos until about 1965 when she retired to Halstead, Essex. She died in 1973. Dr Hubbard was unwilling to discuss her past and despite careful research, very few records have turned up. Her Home Office application for naturalisation as a British citizen is in the National Archives[10] but is currently closed under the Public Records Act. Professor Paul Weindling, at Oxford Brookes University, who has developed a reference collection of over 5000 medical refugees, including 500 Austrians, and wrote an article on those who practised in Wales,[11] had no record of her.[12] Even the WNMA confused her with another refugee, Dr Runhilt von den Steinen-Mayer, who was appointed to North Wales Sanatorium in 1943. Whether from chance or choice, Dr Hubbard seems to have successfully slipped through the nets of officialdom and vanished into legend. In 1947, the sanatorium school passed into the control of the Breaconshire Local Education Authority who appointed a head teacher, Miss Amy White, who had trained at Liverpool University and previously taught at North Wales Sanatorium, Denbigh.[13]

Treatment at Craig-y-nos was still based mainly on fresh air, nourishing food, tonics including iron (which caused constipation and damaged the teeth), artificial pneumothorax (collapse lung therapy), and in some cases, controversial drugs such as sanocrysin (gold therapy). Sanocrysin, with a gold content of about forty per cent, had been discovered in the 1920s and was found to be successful in slowing down the rate at which TB bacteria reproduced. However, it did have side effects associated with metal poisoning such as skin rashes and kidney damage and by the 1940s it was falling out of favour with tuberculosis doctors. Peggy Tizzard (Jones) was treated with gold injections as a child, and Betty Thomas (Dowdle) received fourteen such injections as a twenty-year-old. The first really effective drug (or so-called 'magic bullet') to treat tuberculosis by killing the bacteria that caused it was the antibiotic streptomycin, discovered by Selman Waksman in the United States in 1943, for which he won a Nobel Prize in 1952. Streptomycin did not come to Britain until December 1946, when the Medical Research Council (MRC) in London bought enough to treat 200 people. At that time there was still conflicting evidence about its usefulness in tuberculosis so it was decided to organise a controlled clinical trial – the first of its kind – whereby half of a group of seriously ill patients with pulmonary (lung) TB received streptomycin and bed rest, and the other half received bed rest only. All patients were in the age range fifteen to thirty. After six months, fifty-one per cent of those who had received streptomycin were considerably improved (as judged by chest X-ray) and seven per cent had died. However, in those on bed rest only, twenty-seven per cent had died and just eight per cent had improved.[14] The results were published in 1948 and considered so remarkable that there was soon a black market for streptomycin, and people with private means rushed to buy it directly from America. Dr Thomas Jarman, a very popular doctor with the children of Craig-y-nos, spent a year from 1946-47 touring American tuberculosis hospitals and sent a report about his observations on the new antibiotic to the MRC Streptomycin Committee. In February 1947, he wrote enthusiastically of it to the Principal Medical Officer at the WMNA: 'I am anxious to impress on you that we should fight for the *maximum amount* of Streptomycin we can possibly get, and that we should be included in a liberal way in any streptomycin studies that may be started under MOH (Ministry of Health) or MRC auspices at home.'[15] Although no patients in Craig-y-nos were included in the clinical trial (there were a number from Sully Hospital, Cardiff), it was being used there by 1948. Two of the first to receive it were twelve-year-old Sylvia Floyd (Williams) and Barbara Pye (Dommett) who was eighteen. Barbara was the only person in her ward to have streptomycin and some of the others wondered why and asked for it too. Like all antibiotics, however, streptomycin only worked when the infection was active, that is, when there were tuberculosis bacteria to kill. For people like Barbara, Sylvia, Euryl Thomas, Sylvia Moore (Peckham), and Mary Watkins (Williams), who had active tuberculosis in both lungs and were not expected to survive, streptomycin was literally a life-saver. Its most serious side effect was ear damage, and Pat Hybert (Mogridge) who was given it in 1953 recalled her ears tingling and then completely losing her hearing in one ear.

Within a year of streptomycin's use in Britain, tuberculosis bacteria were becoming resistant to it, a very worrying occurrence. The problem was solved by giving another new drug called para-aminosalicylic acid (PAS) in combination with streptomycin. After 1952, a third drug, isoniazad (Rimifon), was sometimes added. Drug therapy did eventually empty the tuberculosis sanatoria and hospitals but TB doctors, so accustomed to ordering the lives of their incarcerated patients, did not let them go without a fight. A radio programme, *Searchlight on TB*, transmitted on the BBC Welsh Home Service in June 1949, interviewed Dr Watson, the Medical Superintendent of South Wales Sanatorium:

Watson: In spite of all modern advancement the old principles of rest, fresh air, and nutritious food remain the bedrock of all treatment.

J C Griffith Jones (interviewer): You teach patients *when* to rest?
Watson: Not only when to rest but how. So the sanatorium largely becomes a school where the patient is taught a way of life; and that new way of life not only helps towards curing the disease, but also, we hope, provides a guide that will serve patients well for the future.

J C Griffiths: Self discipline counts then?
Watson: To be frank, throughout the period of treatment *and after*, the battle for health must be fought by the patient, even more than by the physician, or surgeon. Without the patient's full co-operation, without educability, self control, steadfastness, and acceptance of a disciplined life on the part of the patient, the whole gamut of treatment may be of little avail. It has been said that no fool was ever cured of tuberculosis; the fool of course being one who does not accept intelligently the ordered life so essential to secure and maintain real betterment.[16]

By the time this programme was broadcast, Craig-y-nos, like other hospitals and sanatoria across Britain was under the control of the newly inaugurated National Health Service. In Wales, hospital services passed to the Welsh Regional Hospital Board and the WNMA was disbanded. Craig-y-nos thus became a NHS hospital.

Children's Stories

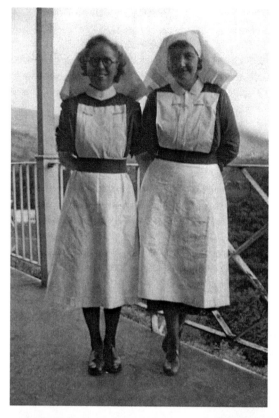

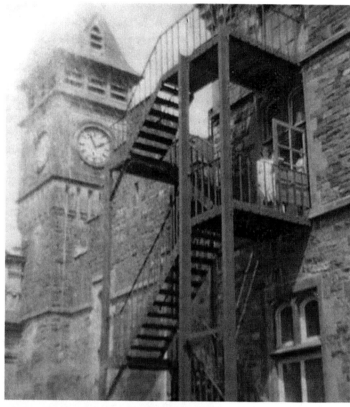

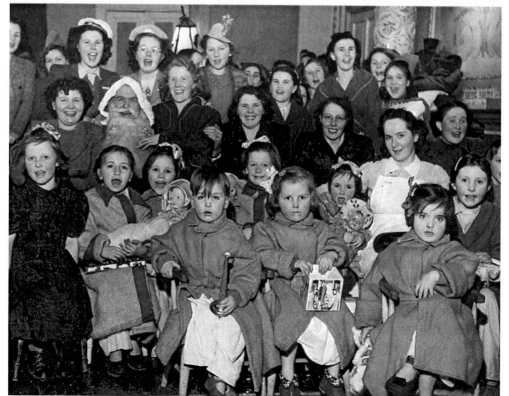

Sister Powell (right), who came to Craig-y-nos in 1936 and was in charge of the Babies' Ward, with Sister Rich. Courtesy Ann Morris.

Long way down. The fire escape outside Ward 2, where the girls would wait for visitors to arrive at two o'clock on the first weekend of the month. Courtesy Christine Perry.

Christmas in Craig-y-nos, 1940s. After a concert in the Adelina Patti theatre, gifts are distributed to the children by Father Christmas, played by Jenkyn Evans, the hospital dentist. The nurse in the photograph is Glenys Jones (Davies). Courtesy Glenys Jones.

Renée Bartlett (Griffiths) - Runaways

I would ask my mum and dad to take me home every time they visited me. It is not that I was mistreated, just that I wanted to be with them. Anyway, I devised a plan to run away from the hospital and I persuaded Lorna, who had been abandoned there and never had any visitors, to come with me.

I used to hear a clock striking the hour at night, and about the same time each night a bus would stop outside. I convinced Lorna we could get on this bus and it would take us home to my mum and dad. I used to watch the nurses each night settling us all down to sleep and turning off the main lights. Sometimes, they would leave the fire escape door open. This one night everything seemed to be going to plan and I tried to make my escape dressed in my pyjamas, dressing gown, and slippers, with my toilet bag in one hand and my doll tucked under my other arm. I persuaded Lorna to follow me. We only got as far as the fire escape before we were caught. I must have caused quite a stir, but the only punishment I remember was being put in a straitjacket and having to explain to my mum and dad when they came next to visit me. It was 1944 and I was six-years-old.

Roger Wyn Beynon – Institutionalised and independent

They found out I had TB when I fell down as a toddler and hurt my right knee. I ended up in Craig-y-nos for five years (1949-54). I remember Coronation Day (1953) there. I remember the peacocks, the park, the train on the far bank, and the (streptomycin) injections - four a day in the bum! As a small child in Craig-y-nos, I missed having a cwtch (cuddle) and buried myself in books. I was always in a book, so I think as an individual I lost myself. The only person I can recall is Graham Canning alongside me. We were bed-bound all the time so I wasn't aware of other children in the ward. Craig-y-nos certainly taught me independence. I was independent in a way that I think anybody who has been institutionalized for a while would be.

I had a brother who was born while I was in hospital so, coming out, I didn't know who he was. I remember coming out of Craig-y-nos and it was a glorious summer's day, and being on the lawn and having all these strange objects coming up to me and making a fuss. I realized afterwards that they were girls, and of course I'd never seen a girl before. I could read and write very well and I found my primary school was rather boring. I was in a caliper until I was about ten. When I had this removed, I had a stern lecture from the doctor about what I could do and what I couldn't do but naturally, being an independent little so-and-so, I ignored them. The only thing I haven't been able to do is to climb trees, and that's mostly to do with the fact that I don't like heights. Certainly I've played sports. The only thing I felt deprived of as a child was that I was unable to ride a bicycle properly. My right leg was sticking out all the time.

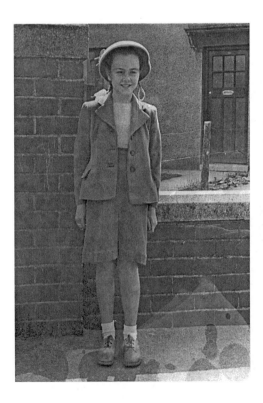
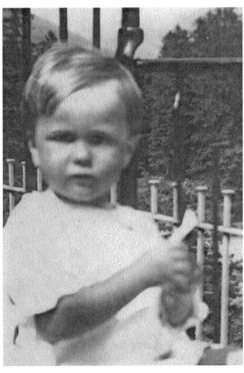

Renée after her discharge from Craig-y-nos. Courtesy Renée Bartlett.

Roger in his cot outside the Babies' Ward. Courtesy Roger Wyn Beynon.

I left grammar school, having passed my exams to join the Royal Navy as an officer. Then I found out that I'd failed my medical as a result of my knee, and that was a real choker. I did become very rebellious with a chip on my shoulder. That wasn't so much at society but towards my parents. I have rheumatoid arthritis. The consultant told me it was inevitable as a result of my experiences as a young boy. I had a replacement knee seven years ago. For the first time in my life, I've got a knee that looks like a knee. The old one looked like a Crunchy Bar and that apparently was a distinct feature of TB in the bone. I know they kept it as a souvenir.

Roger ran his own engineering business until 1998. He is married to a psychologist who wrote her thesis on institutionalization.

John Nelson - Just an empty, unmade bed

I was nine at the time, in 1947. My mother and I travelled to Craig-y-nos from Cardiff and it took all day, with the final leg of the journey on a bus from Swansea. The ward I was in was just inside the balcony - plenty of fresh air inside and I was not envious of those out on the balcony. Their lives must have been hell in the winter, beds covered with a tarpaulin to save the bedding getting wet! I would suggest that their lives were shortened by this primitive ('cruel'?) treatment. It's more like death by misadventure. We were allowed onto the balcony and we would chat to those in bed. Sometimes, the person you had been talking to one day was not there the next day - just an empty unmade bed. This happened too many times. It was a scary lesson to learn for someone of a tender age.

I have no bad impressions of my stay at the castle. The medical treatments were usual for the time and one can see now that they were rather primitive by the standards of today. The only regret I have now is that I cannot recall having any schoolwork at all. I later failed my eleven-plus and I always put this down to this gap in my education. The question that has always intrigued me is the psychological effect of being parted from family and friends for such a long time, the strain on parents of having a child such a long distance away out of their control, and the long-term effect on the young immature patients. Visiting for my parents meant a long day's travel from Cardiff plus fares, and they certainly were not rich. After fifteen months at the castle I was moved to Highland Moors, Llandrindod Wells, spending another nine months convalescing.

TB is a great nuisance. After about six years it came back to annoy me for another two years - eighteen months in Talgarth (the South Wales Sanatorium) and then a little visit to Sully Hospital, near Cardiff, where they snipped out the naughty TB from my right lung. I enjoyed it at the seaside - it was warmer than the Swansea Valley!

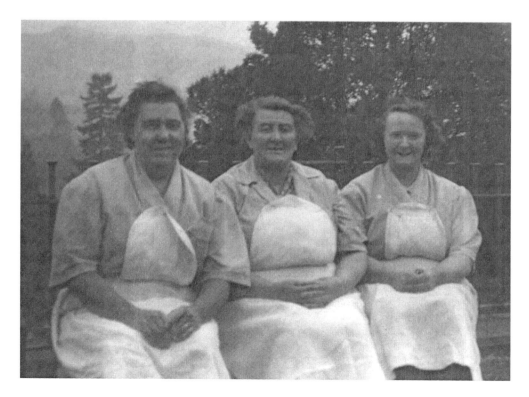

Domestic staff were less authoritarian than medical and nursing staff, and would sometimes sneak in sweets and comics for the children. Courtesy of Peggy Jones.

Caroline Boyce (Havard) - No system of education

I can remember being taken, aged nine, to the doctor with shiny lesions on my shins, diagnosed as erythema nodosum, indicating that infections are present in the body. TB was diagnosed. My mother cried and I felt very helpless and confused. It was 1949. I was put in the top floor children's ward (girls only), with windows overlooking the front courtyard and main road. There was a large wooden table in the middle of the room where we ate meals once we were allowed out of bed. There were no pictures on the walls, no curtains on the windows – only iron bars - no flowers or plants. The floor was shiny brown and was polished by a quiet, pleasant woman called Annie, wearing a pink and white striped overall. She had a large tin of liquid polish, which she placed in dollops on the floor before attacking it with a buffer hinged on a long handle.

My treatment revolved around bed rest and eating, although the only food I can remember is porridge, which I hated. It was grey and contained crunchy bits. We were allowed up in stages, starting with half an hour a day. At two hours we were allowed to wear day clothes, a great excitement. I was a bit too active when I was first up. I remember dancing and singing, and my temperature shot up. I was put back on full bed rest. I remember the feeling of companionship in the wards. I always enjoyed being able to go to the ward below to visit the older girls, including an acquaintance from Brecon, Mary Davies (now Slater), and Ann Rumsey (now Shaw), whose mother sometimes gave my mother a lift to the hospital on visiting days. We would stand at the windows waiting for the visitors to arrive and would wave and call to them before they were allowed in at two pm. I envied the girls on the balcony. Although exposed to the elements, they seemed much freer and had wide panoramic views of the surrounding countryside. Walking with a group of girls in the grounds was a special delight.

The staff varied. Dr Williams (the Medical Superintendent) was a kind of god, Dr Hubbard was terrifying, Sister Morgan stern but kind. One nurse I remember with mixed feelings was Betty Rowe. I was frightened of spiders, and one day she put a dead one in my bed. She talked about Adelina Patti's ghost wandering the castle corridors, which fed my terror of the plaster room. It was a big walk-in closet where unused plaster beds were stored upright. In the gloom they looked like large, misshapen figures. Whenever I had to pass the room I would hope that the door would be shut, and if it was open, run (which was forbidden) past as quickly as I could. There were two teachers, wearing blue overalls, who appeared from time to time with sheets of simple sums and a choice of books. There appeared to be no plan or system of education, and the little work we did was collected without comment and never returned. I remember doing a lot of drawing, reading anything I could get my hands on, and writing letters and stories. We experienced long periods of endless boredom. At Christmas, I recall being uncomfortably aware that I had more parcels than some children, particularly Sybil, a travellers' child with dark unruly hair and very dark brown eyes. The day they brought her in was terrifying. She cried miserably and her parents stood at the door weeping, reluctant to leave her. They had a strong smell of wood smoke about them.

When I was discharged I missed the company of the other children and felt lonely at home. My parents bought me a radio and this established a listening habit which has never left me. Although I passed the eleven-plus to Brecon Girls Grammar School, I only just scraped in. I found the discipline and routine of a formal grammar school education difficult to accept after many months of sparse, poor quality schooling. I can understand other ex-patients when they say that they were 'a bit of a loner', 'emotionally vulnerable, but self-reliant' upon discharge. I felt a certain dislocation from my family, who I think found me 'difficult' when I returned home. The whole experience turned me into quite a detached person for many years, and sad though it sounds, I think that for the remainder of my childhood I expected everything and nothing from adults - a good coping strategy.

I trained as an occupational therapist in Oxford. After marriage and two children I retrained and became a teacher. I combined the two disciplines and taught children with two categories of special needs, cerebral palsy and autism. It is easy, looking back, to see where the roots of this career path lie.

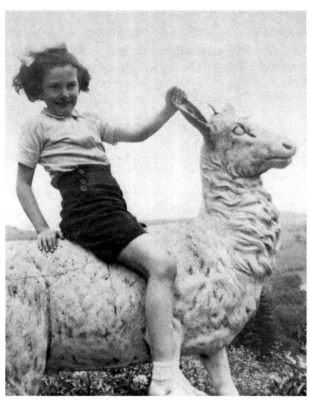
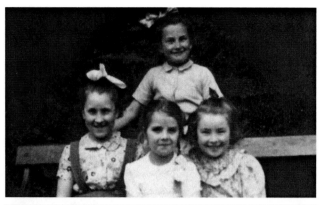
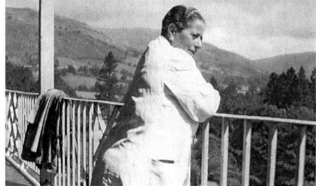

Douglas Herbert - Force-fed cabbage

I was restrained on many occasions. They had this contraption, which had material across the chest and four straps. One strap was tied to the lower right, one to the upper right, and the same on the left. No matter how hard I tried I couldn't get those knots! Because it was the war years, food was scarce. We used to get things like fresh farm eggs. I remember them bringing in an apple or two and on one occasion an orange. I don't recall having much fruit. One of the things I couldn't stand, and can't now, is cabbage. I used to be force-fed cold cabbage. The nurse would bring a bowl along at the same time so that I could be sick into it. There was a lot of iron medicine and we were fed regular doses of syrup of figs because the iron medicine would constipate you. We were given a bedpan every morning. They woke you up at six o'clock and you didn't get breakfast until you used it. If you were constipated that was really something else. I didn't have a lot of treatment except the tube down the throat (gastric lavage). It takes me ten minutes to swallow an aspirin now.

I remember the 1947 Derby Day. I had forty-seven visitors clustered around my bed because mine was the only workable radio. My father had put a sixpenny bet each way on 'My Love' and it won. A couple of years ago there was this pub quiz - a free pint of beer to anyone who could tell them the winner of the 1947 Derby. I put my hand up. My father was astonished because he knew I had no interest in horses. So I reminded him of that day in Craig-y-nos. We had this doctor. She was Austrian, short, and dare I say it, 'little Hitler' gone mad. On one occasion the boys made paper aeroplanes and we were throwing them around. One landed on the floor and I went to get it even though it was 'Silence Hour'. As I did so, she came in and said, 'In bed for a fortnight!' I thought evil thoughts of her. The matron was always for the children. She used to give the staff hell. There was one nurse, a redhead that stuck in my mind. She was fabulous. Nothing was too much trouble and she would even sing you a lullaby. On the day my parents came to take me home they brought me a small jigsaw and I gave it to my friend Andrew in the next bed. His back was encased in plaster of Paris. He had TB of the spine. Six weeks after I left I was told he had died. I was devastated.

As a young man, not long married, we had a group of friends around to our flat. They got out this Ouija board. I didn't want to play so I sat across the living room. I had never talked about Craig-y-nos. I had never discussed with my wife what had gone on in hospital, and it started: 'Does anybody know Andrew?' I said he had been a child with me but I wouldn't discuss it. I wrote on a bit of paper: 'What was the last thing I gave Andrew?' They spelled out 'Jigsaw'. Nobody at that table knew. I asked what was on his back and they spelled out 'Plaster.'

Douglas works as an accountant in Swansea.

Lynette Davies (Evans) – Deprived of a toy

The ward was directly in front of the front door with cots all the way round and windows behind. We were in the cots all the time. Once, I stood up in the cot to shut a window because the other children were asking, and was being punished for it. After that, when all the toys came around, I wasn't allowed a toy, and they did that to other children too. You were bypassed if you had been naughty or you'd said or done something. The dishing out of the toys was the highlight of the day. It was wartime (1941) and people in our village, Aberdare, shared their (ration) coupons so that my parents could bring me sweets and fruit. My mother and father cycled to Craig-y-nos once a month. My grandfather cycled as well. It's a long, long way, and it's not flat.

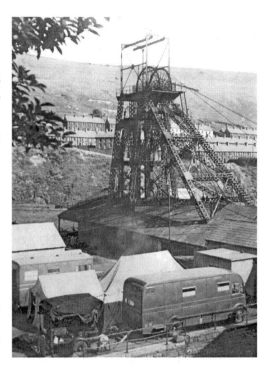

I remember a treatment room and the smell of rubber pipes being put into my throat (gastric lavage). I can smell that rubber now. It frightens me. There was a men's ward and when I was out and about I was sent into that room to pick up all the paper and the rubbish, and put it in a bag. I was only five. My mother never told me that I had TB. I was about fifteen when found I had it. The mobile X-ray came around the workplace, I went for an X-ray and they sent a letter to my mother saying I had scarring on my lung. I couldn't have any children, so I adopted two. They said it was because of the TB. The disease damaged my fallopian tubes. Some women were told they couldn't adopt because they had TB as a child. They never asked so I never told them.

I realize now that there were a lot of quite cruel aspects to Craig-y-nos. They did things that wouldn't now be considered acceptable, like not giving you a toy to play with. The crime was nothing. You then were sitting in a cot all day long with no toy. That's deprivation - terrible when you think of it.

Pat O'Byrne (Mathoulin) – Lost little souls

My father, a miner, died of TB meningitis in 1945. My sister and I were X-rayed and I had TB. I was five. My mother announced that I was going to spend a few days with my Auntie Renée, whom I had only seen on one occasion. My auntie's 'amazing' house was, in fact, Craig-y-nos. Later, my mother told me, 'I *had* to get you into hospital.' So, she did it that way, which was horrific. By that evening, I had adapted. The following morning, no trouble, no sound, everything was alright. There's nothing explained to you at all. We were so controlled. When I woke up in the middle of the night, wanting to go to the toilet, I couldn't go because I knew I had to go down this horrific corridor in this castle, and I was frightened. Oh, I was in agony wanting to go to the toilet and I was petrified to go. I can remember one stormy night being *absolutely* petrified. Thunder and lightening, and the rain lashing on those windows of the Glass Conservatory. You could see into the great rolling clouds.

We had little brown tunic tops and shorts. Our hair was cut almost above our ears in a basin crop so we all looked alike. We had to be fattened up, of course, and for breakfast there was always fried bread brought around on a huge aluminium platter. By the time it came to me it was almost cold. I didn't see china for twenty-two months. My mother would bring me a few sweets and they would be confiscated with all the other children's sweets. We wouldn't eat them ourselves. That would be so greedy. I also remember my mother bringing me a beautiful china doll for Christmas, yet it wasn't mine because we had to learn to share. If another little child wanted to hold that doll or take it to bed, then I would have her teddy bear, and that's how it was. I share everything to this day, even though I want it myself.

But when I got home from hospital, I cried. I wanted to go back. I missed my friends *so* much. Children who had TB had to have a room of their own, and the window would be open every night. My mother put me in cotton wool. I couldn't go to the cinema. I couldn't go dancing. She was *petrified* of TB. When I went back to school, and of course it was a small village (Seven Sisters), I was told not to discuss it at all. 'Where have you been?' 'Oh, I've been on holiday.' 'What happened to your father?' 'He died in the war.' My mother died ten years ago. She would be horrified to know I've talked about Craig-y-nos. But it's always there. I can't ever really forget it, and because of all the attention I got as a child after being there I've worried about my health throughout my life.

Pat married and left Wales at the age of eighteen. She became a shorthand-typist and lives in Yorkshire.

Pat O'Byrne (Mathoulin)
– Shadows of my past

Pat composed this poem after she'd made contact with
The Children of Craig-y-nos project in the summer of 2007.

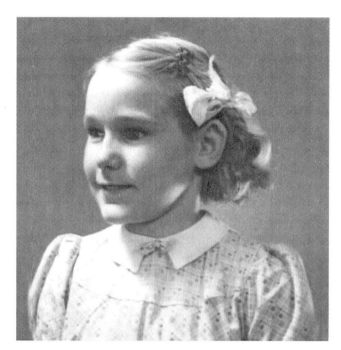

We were those children that you speak of today,
But why weren't we spoken of then?

As each of us languished in beds that were cold
Wondering what tomorrow would bring.

Would we be frightened once more of 'that tube'
And would our hands be restrained by a nurse?

Would our mothers be there to calm our fears
And support us in our distress?

No! For our mothers had left us a long time ago,
And no-one had understood why.

And as we fought inner conflicts with a spirit so brave
We had dreams without any good-byes.

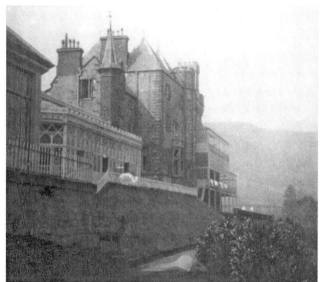

We knew nothing of happiness, or of love,
And knew nothing of what really was wrong.

We were lost little souls who had been left so alone
Until that monthly visit came along.

The sanatorium is now no more,
The lucky ones are healed and gone,
But the scars that are left will never be healed
For they'll just go on and on.

Opposite page

Medical Research Council mobile
mass X-ray vehicle parked beneath
a pit head at Tylorstown, Rhondda
Valley, *c.*1949. Courtesy Cardiff
University, Cochrane Archive,
University Hospital Llandough.

Above

Pat after she had left
Craig-y-nos. Courtesy
Pat O'Byrne.

Craig-y-nos Castle depicted
here as the impregnable
fortress that so many of the
children considered it to be.
Courtesy Dulcie Oltersdorf.

Peter Wagstaffe – Nightlines in the river

Most of the time, I was in a splint with my legs apart and straps across my chest. You could only move your head and arms. I was on the balcony all the time (1940-45) apart from a fortnight over Christmas. We used to make up our own games. We were in a row in beds and we used to play cricket. We'd have a book on one locker - that was the wicket, and we'd have a patient about three beds away with a big ball of newspaper rolled up on a string. He'd bowl the ball to us and try to hit the wicket, and if we could hit it the length of four beds, it was four runs, and six beds it was six runs. The girls in the ward up above used to drop string down with notes for us, and we'd send notes up to them. Once we were taken to Swansea beach for the day by bus. Those that couldn't walk were carried. Our parents got to know about it and they were all down on the beach waiting for us.

After I had been there about five years Dr Hubbard arrived. She walked with a limp herself. As soon as she came, she said, 'Get him up, get him up!' Then we - the children with TB hips - were up and home in about six months. I wonder how long I'd have been there if she hadn't come. Those boys who were allowed up could walk around the grounds. They had fishing lines brought in by their parents, and they'd lay nightlines in the river going through the grounds. They'd go down in the morning, and the fish they'd caught at the end of the lines the staff would cook for the patients who were pretty ill. Quite a few boys died and some were on the balcony with me. One boy was covered in abscesses. He went home to die. One evening, there were a few American soldiers walking around the grounds and we all shouted, 'Have you got any gum chum?' They said, 'We'll be back tomorrow night,' and they did come back with sweets, chocolates and gum. They were from the military training camp at Sennybridge in the Brecon Beacons.

Going home again was lovely, beautiful. There were no problems adjusting. I had a caliper on when I came out of Craig-y-nos but I had to go back after about six months to have my hip locked (this is called arthrodesis and results in a completely stiff joint). I've got a nasty curvature of the spine.

Peter worked for forty years in the Treasurer's Department of the National Health Service in Neath and Swansea.

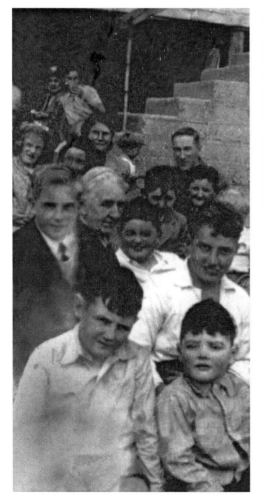

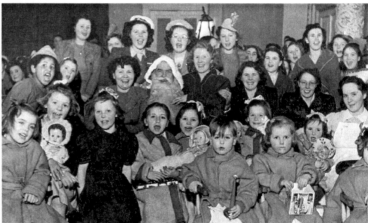

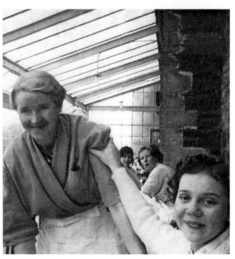

Day out at Swansea beach, early 1940s. Peter is the boy in the centre, sitting next to his grandmother. Courtesy Peter Wagstaffe.

Christmas in Craig-y-nos, 1940s. After a concert in the Adelina Patti theatre, gifts are distributed to the children by Father Christmas, played by Jenkyn Evans, the hospital dentist. The nurse in the photograph is Glenys Jones (Davies). Courtesy Glenys Jones.

Miss Rees, a domestic, was popular with the children. Courtesy Christine Perry.

Rose Pugh (Hunt) - Afraid to sleep

Even to this day I don't sleep very well because I was afraid to go to sleep in Craig-y-nos. The nurses used to say, 'Oh she died in her sleep.' I used to think, 'Well, I don't want to die', and I would struggle to keep awake. In the wards you could hear the groans and the moans and the coughing and the spitting, and the ones that were out on the veranda were those that weren't so bad. My uncle was in the Navy and he was allowed to come in with a hand of bananas. Each banana was cut in half and there were just enough to go round so there must have been close on twenty in the ward. Everybody would pass me their porridge because it was thick with lumps and there was me pushing it down the waste pipe on the veranda, and one day it rained so heavy the porridge all bubbled back up. There were a couple of ladies who came in from outside - they were cleaners - absolutely marvellous. They used to bring in comics and sneak in sweets. I suppose the nurses had a job to do but some were bitches. Some took great delight in tucking you in so tight in bed that you couldn't move. Others were absolutely lovely.

On one visit my mother missed the bus and she was crying at the bus stop. A Post Office van pulled up and he put my mother in the back with the mailbags and dropped her at Craig-y-Nos. I can remember my mother turning up at my sixth birthday, 3rd May, and my sister was born on the 7th. The baker's in Swansea High Street was very, very good and when my mother told him that it was my birthday he sent up trifles. He made the trifles in waxed cartons - this was 1941 - but when my mother arrived they were running everywhere. Ralph, 'the books' in Swansea used to give my mother comics that had been damaged so she would turn up laden.

I blocked out my experience at Craig-y-Nos. Up until last year I used to do talks in schools and women's groups about being an evacuee. It was appalling, and I think that's where I got my TB. I wasn't evacuated far but the family didn't want us and I had to sleep in a cabin trunk. We literally didn't get food. The man had a constant cough. They said it was because he had been a miner but the idea of my mother, later, was that he had TB and that's where I picked it up. Craig-y-nos definitely had an effect on me. It made me a much stronger person. I'm not afraid to travel on my own. I'm not afraid to face things.

Sylvia Floyd (Williams) - Five Christmases in Craig-y-nos

Craig-y-nos may have been a wonderful castle in magnificent grounds with views of the Brecon Beacons but I was eleven-years-old, very ill, and miles from home and my mother. It was 1947. For the next four years I was confined to bed, not allowed to go to the bathroom or the toilet. Many girls in my ward where sent home to die. I had five cavities in my lungs, and in 1948, had to have part of my lung removed in Morriston Hospital. Every week for the next three and a half years I had Artificial Pneumothorax (collapse of the lung). A thick needle was inserted between my ribs on my left side, to go through to my lung. It was attached to a pipe and air was pressed into my lung. Dr Hubbard was a very harsh woman - Austrian. I dare not think about shedding a tear or crying while she did this painful procedure.

Every Sunday my mother took a brown carrier bag to Swansea bus station and paid two shillings for a ticket for that bag to travel on the bus to Craig-y-nos. I could watch from the window and see the bus driver bring my brown paper carrier bag into the hospital. Every week my mother would be sending sweets, chocolates and half a dozen eggs, which the nurses would cook for my breakfast or mix up into a glass of milk (long before the days of salmonella, of course). I might have new pyjamas or maybe new slippers. Always a book. I felt very lucky. We had lovely staff nurse, Glenys Davies. She did everything in her power to make us happy. Sister Morgan was our ward sister; Auntie Maggie was ward auxiliary nurse. There was no television in those days, and every Sunday night Sister Morgan allowed us to listen to Donald Peers. He played music similar to top of the pops, I would think. I spent five Christmases in Craig-y-Nos and every year my mother would a fill a large suitcase with presents and goodies, and in the middle of the night the nurse would put every case by the side of every girl's bed. Father Christmas (Jenkyn Evans, the hospital dentist) would come on Christmas Day and we all had a gift. Dr Williams (the Medical Superintendent) came to each ward to carve the turkey on the table.

The boy's ward was immediately below us and I used to send notes tied to a piece of string over the balcony to Godfrey Boniface. I considered him to be my very first boyfriend. In actual fact, I don't think I ever saw him. I used to shout to him over the balcony. I remember Miss Thomas (the teacher) had me enter a hand-writing competition, and I won a Conway Stuart fountain pen. At the time, I had pen pals all over the world. One was in Australia and she would send me a parcel of tinned fruit. It was wonderful. I don't think we could have had tinned fruit in the hospital in those days. I shared it with the others in the ward but always saved a tin for my mother to take home. During my five years in Ward 2 I am not going to say they were 'the happiest days of my life', far from it, but they were not miserable days either. We were all in the same boat, all missing our families. Streptomycin came in and I was one of the first patients to be given it. It saved my life. On the final 'Long Round' Dr Williams told me they were going to send me home. I wrote to my mother in huge letters across the page: 'I CAN COME HOME'. I was sixteen.

Myra Elizabeth Rees (Thomas) - No sad thoughts

I'm one of nine children, and after my older sister (aged fifteen) died of TB in 1943, we were all tested. I was so puny and ill-looking that they took me into hospital for observation. I was seven. My father took me on the bus to Craig-y-nos. They searched my hair for nits then put me to bed and I remember crying for my mother. I can't remember anyone being nasty and I have no sad thoughts about being in Craig-y-nos. I was there a year, then a year and a half in Llanybyther (West Wales Sanatorium).

There was a little bit of a stigma when I started school again. They put me to sit by this girl who lived not far from me, and her mother objected to me sitting next to her. I always remember that.

Myra has since enjoyed good health and is a great-grandmother.

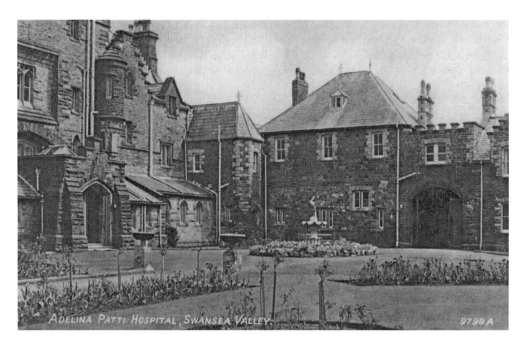

In this view of Craig-y-nos, the main entrance door is left, whilst the buildings behind the fountain (centre) housed the X-ray and light therapy rooms, operating theatre and dental department. From an old postcard.

Terry Hunt - Restrainers

I picked TB up from my uncle. He served with my father in the Merchant Navy during the war. My uncle had a rough campaign and when he came out he was quite ill. He lived with us for some time and used to play with me when I was a small boy. He was the classic TB sufferer - very, very thin, white skinned, and never ran anywhere. He just did odd jobs, and he lived in a Haig Home all the time I knew him, and of course in those days, people smoked whether they had TB or not. I went into Craig-y-nos for a year as a seven-year-old in 1947, followed by another at Highland Moors (Llandrindod Wells).

The feeling I had in Craig-y-nos was almost one of helplessness, that you couldn't do anything. I found it boring there. I was in straitjackets but I remember breaking out of them and having heavier ones put on me to tie me down to the bed. When somebody stood over you to make sure you never got out of bed, you can either treat it as for your own good or see that person as a jailer. When I told my parents things that had happened, like having your sweets taken away and being tied to the bed, they just didn't believe me. It was a case of, 'Oh, he's always telling stories, always telling lies.' I always thought my parents didn't come to see me very often because they didn't want to or they couldn't afford to. It would have made a difference if I had known that visiting was only allowed once a month.

I found grammar school quite a struggle and I found sports activities a tremendous effort. The gym teacher made me run around the gym and I was absolutely exhausted. When he was asking me why I couldn't do it, I started trying to tell him that I'd been in a sanatorium for two years and he said, 'Stop making excuses,' and he smacked my backside. Now I've grown up I don't tell people about it. When I was a kid, the other children in the street weren't allowed to play with me. You're not to go too close to them in case you're infectious. In my early thirties, when I was still playing rugby, if I went in for an X-ray, I was always whipped down the chest clinic to be checked over. I struggled in education until I was about eighteen, and then I started catching up. I qualified as a metallurgist through day release and studying at night school.

On the day my parents came to take me home they brought me a small jigsaw and I gave it to my friend Andrew in the next bed. His back was encased in plaster of Paris. He had TB of the spine.

Six weeks after I left I was told he had died.

I was devastated.

Douglas Herbert

Roy Harry - Gastric lavage

I didn't have breakfast this morning, something to do with a test. Maybe I could have breakfast later. I thought having a test was someone opening my pyjama top and listening to my chest and my back. This was very different.

A nurse came to get me. She held my hand and we walked out of Ward 1 along the corridor, the same corridor along which I had made my bid for freedom when my mother had left me in the hospital. There were two or three doors along the right side and we went through one of these. I was sat on a chair facing a window, the door directly behind me. I was aware of another nurse doing something with a rubber tube. I think they explained what was about to happen but I don't remember what they said. One nurse was holding me, telling me to open my mouth; the other one trying to hold my chin down whilst she pushed the tube into my mouth. This caused me to panic. I shook my head violently, kicked my feet out as hard as I could, repeatedly, until I was sliding down the seat of the chair. The tube thing was put aside and I was repositioned in the chair. They were going to have another go.

Between my crying and sobs I was begging them not to do it again. They didn't listen, of course, so now I was held really firmly. Once again, the tube entered my mouth. I mustered up every ounce of strength to continue my struggle, the tube reached the back of my throat and I heaved as though I would be sick. I had to stop it going down. I bit hard onto the tube which halted its progress. I could taste tears which had run into my mouth. The nurse in charge of the tube-pushing shouted at me. She said if I bit through it I could die. The words terrified me but I couldn't bring myself to release my grip on it. I felt the grip on my arms slacken and the one holding me down said, 'Go and fetch Sister Powell.' I was crying bitterly.

The end was surprisingly quick. Sister Powell arrived. She was barking rather than talking. 'What's all this fuss? I won't stand for it.' Now there were two holders and one formidable tube operator. The tube went down and I went rigid, trembling and shivering from head to toe. Seconds later it was all over. Soon I was back in my bed in Ward 1.

Roy's first experience of a gastric lavage, aged three and a half, in 1945.

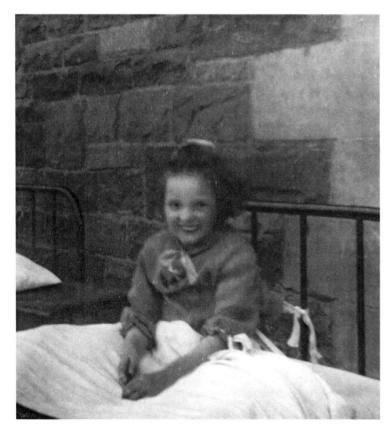

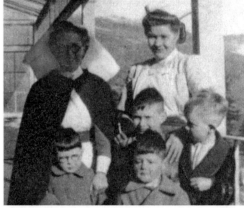

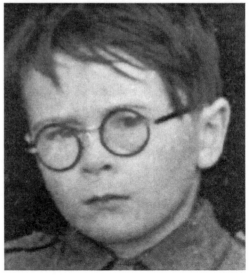

Child tied to the bed in a restraining jacket. The children called them 'straitjackets'. Courtesy Norma Lewis.

Roy (left with glasses) on Ward 1 balcony, 1945. Courtesy Peter Wagstaffe.

Roy after his discharge from Craig-y-nos. Courtesy Roy Harry.

Gwyn Thomas – Diphtheria carrier

I cried like crazy and my father was very traumatized by leaving me in Craig-y-nos. My mother had been unwilling to let me go because she believed that everybody who went there died. She tried to reverse the doctor's decision. It was 1942 and I was six-years-old. As a consequence of my TB, our family did not have to have an evacuee billeted with them during the war. I did not realize until speaking to my father years later that they were only allowed to visit once a month on Sundays from 2-4 pm. However, a local minister was allowed to visit at any time and brought me grapes. I was only there for seven months because I was found to be a diphtheria carrier and was transferred to Tonnach, an isolation hospital. There, my parents were not allowed to visit me at all. The only way they could find out if I was dead or alive was through the local newspaper that carried an account each week of how patients were progressing.

The Craig-y-nos experience did me no harm – it made me tough as nails. I couldn't write when I went there so somebody wrote a letter to my mother for me. I returned to Craig-y-nos twice as a visitor when I was forty. It had been converted to a hospital for elderly people. On my second visit I was shown my medical records and X-rays. In my notes I found a letter from my mother to me, which I had never been given. I took it and still have it.

I was the first doctor in the family and met my wife at medical school. My son, nephew and brother are also doctors. I have always talked freely with my family of my experiences at Craig-y-nos.

Gwyn lives in Norfolk.

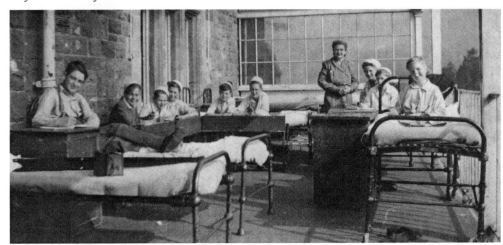

Boys having lessons on the balcony of Ward 1 with the headmistress, Miss Amy White. There was no facility for isolating children with acute infectious diseases like diphtheria because Craig-y-nos was always overcrowded. Courtesy Mari Friend.

Jean Hopkins (Phillips) - An outbreak of diphtheria

I was admitted to Craig-y-nos at the age of eleven with a TB gland. It was 1942. I had sun-ray treatment and was never confined to bed. I was the oldest child on the ward. All our crockery and cutlery were numbered. This enabled each patient to have the same set each mealtime. I was number 44. No children (under sixteen) were allowed in as visitors, so for nine months I did not see my three brothers and little sister who was five-years-old. One disastrous occurrence was an outbreak of diphtheria on our ward. We were all swabbed and the infected patients were transferred to the isolation hospital. One of our nicest nurses went with them. Whether she contracted the disease or just went as their nurse I never knew.

A new patient introduced us to her hobby of writing to film stars for an autographed photograph. I became very keen on this and was soon in receipt of my first one, Gene Autry and his horse Trigger. My time was spent reading, doing jigsaws and knitting. One idiotic rule I can remember was no knitting on a Sunday. We had a nurse and domestic from the Bible College. The nurse would teach us religious songs, which we sang to Dr Jarman, whom we all adored. He was not amused, as he expected a more lively and cheerful singsong. He must have had a word with Sister, as we never repeated that performance. Sister Morgan was very kind. On one occasion she took a few of us blackberry picking. We crossed the river over the little bridge and had a very enjoyable afternoon. Sister assured us we would be the first to sample the tart as soon as cook had made it. She would take me to the Patti theatre on the promise I would not tell the other children. I only ever saw Deanna Durbin films.

A parcel arrived from my teacher in Terrace Road School, Miss Rowe. It contained bars of chocolate donated by the girls in Standard Five. When you consider it was wartime and sweets were rationed, this was an incredible gesture by these young girls. Of course, the parcel was whisked away, and the content shared amongst us all. Whilst lying in bed at night, I was aware of the bombing raids. I could hear the explosions quite clearly. My thoughts were instantly of my family in Swansea.

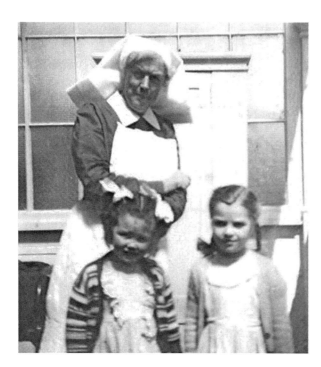

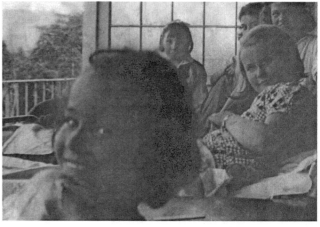

Sister Winnie Morgan with two little girls. Sister Morgan came to Craig-y-nos in 1923 as a Staff Nurse and was promoted to Sister the following year. She remained until retirement in the mid-1950s. Courtesy Ann Shaw.

Christine (near left) in her balcony bed with friends. Courtesy Christine Thornton.

Christine Thornton (Davies) - Balcony in the snow

Our house in Swansea was bombed and we were evacuated to the outskirts of the city. I was one of nine children. My father died in 1943, a year before I went to Craig-y-nos, aged nearly seven, with TB hip. Dr Hubbard examined my legs and I remember screaming with pain because she couldn't straighten my right leg. I was put on to an iron A-frame. It was difficult for some parts of my body to be washed and despite being rubbed with methylated spirits I did get bedsores and I still have the scars today. The doctor told my mother I might not survive but I did make progress and eventually I was put into a plaster cast that covered my right leg and my body to under my arms. Then I had a caliper fitted from ankle to thigh on my right leg. I was twenty-four before I could walk without the caliper.

We were on the balcony in the snow of 1947. The nurses were wonderful although they must have been freezing. They put Vaseline on our faces to stop them chapping. We had green tarpaulins on the bed to keep off the rain and snow. I couldn't snuggle down because I was rigid in this frame so I would pull the covers over my face for warmth. The cold was the best cure for TB in those days. In order to eat I had to balance the food on my chest and I could just raise my head enough to feed myself. Once we went to see a show in Swansea. They put a board over two or three seats on the bus and my iron frame was laid on to this board. Another time I remember going to Swansea Bay. People gathered around us just looking and smiling. Anything new brought in had to be fumigated first. I didn't have much schooling because I was on an iron frame. I was taught how to knit so my doll had some clothes.

I was put into a D class when I went back to school. I knew very little because of the number of years that I hadn't had schooling, but determination gave me the will to learn and I was in an A class when I left at fifteen. I was restricted as to what work I could do. My right hip was completely fused, my shoe was raised by two inches, and the muscles in this leg were wasted. I was registered disabled. I worked in Mettoys in Swansea, sitting all day assembling toys, but I was admitted to Craig-y-nos again in 1952 with TB in my lungs. I was in the 'Six Bedder' (Adelina Patti's bedroom). We played 'I spy' and once we had a séance at midnight. We all got out of bed for this and the screeching of the glass across the glass-topped table frightened us so much we never did again. One girl did die and it was a very sad time for us. We often teased the nurses and they got their own back by giving us cold bedpans, which were made of steel in those days. Once we had finished our course of streptomycin, which took about nine months, we were allowed to get up each day.

Despite my loss of schooling and the lifelong disability of my TB hip, I did manage to learn a lot and ended up doing some really good jobs including security and floor work as a store detective. Nobody expected a lame woman to be a detective!

My health has deteriorated over the past twenty-five years. I have had my TB hip rebuilt and replaced; also my left knee has been replaced. My spine is also quite bad, and I have a lung disease. I still get around. I use two arm crutches for walking but my mobility is very limited. As for emotional and psychological support in those days, well there was none! You were left to get on with it. My memories of Craig-y-nos are mostly happy ones, and I am still in awe of the place every time I see it.

Maureen Powell - Take me home

Maureen composed this poem in 1942, age ten. She did not know that she had TB. Later, the children of Craig-y-nos amended it to *The TB flushes* and set it to music.

I had the scarlet fever,
I had it very bad.
They wrapped me up in a blanket
And put me in a van,
The van was very shaky,
I nearly did fall out
And when I reached the hospital
I heard a patient shout:

'Mammy, Daddy take me home
from this hospital
I want to be home with you.'

Here comes the nurse
With a red hot poker,
Drops it down
And takes no notice.

'Oh,' said the patient,
'That's too hot.'
'Oh,' said the nurse,
'I am sure it's not.'

They tied you to a cabbage stalk
And cut me up with a knife and fork.

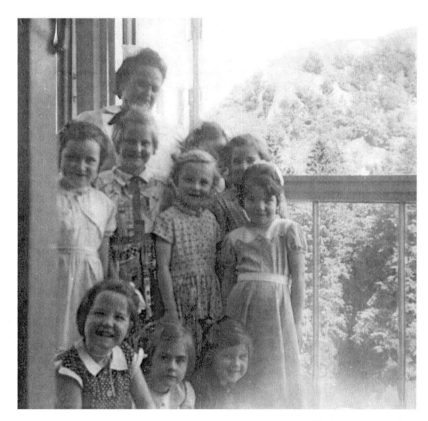

Singing was a popular pastime at Craig-y-nos, both formally and informally. Courtesy Christine Perry.

Vera Blewett (Paris) - The family secret

My father was away fighting in the war and my mother died of TB in March 1942, and then they found that I had it too. I was only about three-years-old when I was in Craig-y-nos. I was institutionalized for a year and eight months instead of being with a family. That has an effect on you for the rest of your life. When I was about seventeen I found out that my father had remarried after my mother's death and the mother I had wasn't my real mother. Within a few months of my finding out this big family secret, my father died.

Many years ago I went to Craig-y-nos with a group of people. I told someone that I was a child there. Perhaps there'd be some photographs hidden away that I could have a look at, but the man I spoke to said, 'No, we don't talk about that.' Later, I was showing a photo of me as a child in Craig-y-nos to a dear friend, a retired nurse, when she said, 'I know that nurse. She used to work in Swansea General Hospital.' And she was holding me in the photograph! I was told that when I came out of hospital, the thing I loved doing most was sitting on the stairs singing hymns. The nurse that my friend pointed out, apparently, was very religious. So there's no doubt that whilst I was in Craig-y-nos, she taught us hymns.

It's a part of my life when I was very young that I really know nothing about. Maybe I was searching for my missing past - and I still am.

Robert Evans (Allsopp) - Isolation, cruelty and kindness

The memories of Craig-y-nos never leave me, for they are the formative experiences of my life - the six-year-old coughing and wasting away, with his sister Judy in a ward nearby but removed from her brother's sight. In the scheme of life in South Wales, consumption's finger touched six of our family, killing three. Those first months were not pleasant. I became withdrawn, trying to avoid upsetting the staff. I was humiliated by my bed-wetting, which I tried to hide by various stratagems, all of them futile. I was so withdrawn that I cannot remember the name of any other patient during my time there.

I do remember Santa Claus entertaining us in the Patti theatre. He was my uncle, Jenkyn Evans from Ystalyfera, a dentist by profession and a sculptor of some note by avocation. Sister Jones stayed in my mind for years as an object of fear, always in a snit with a viper's tongue and contempt for children. I watched a programme on television about the fight for women's suffrage in Britain. Many of the imprisoned demonstrators went on hunger-strike, only to be force-fed, yes! Through conical glass funnels and red rubber tubes. I was transported back in time to a side-ward in Craig-y-nos, to being tortured by four women, a glass funnel and a red rubber tube. The terrifying 'tube days' survive, indelible as tattoos in my head.

For sixty years I have wondered why a party of children was allowed to roam the grounds without an adult in attendance. For adventurers there is always danger, in this case in the form of a deep, square pool, into which, too curious by half, one boy fell, unable to swim. Somebody ran for help, and the others managed to reach me, struggling with an imaginary breast-stroke. A nurse took me back to the hospital. She put me in a hot deep bath, where she dunked my head underwater again and again to rid me of my dread.

Surely there was no conscious cruelty. The staff must have been practising the 'best practice' of 1946 and 47. If they did not explain that to me, well, that too, was what doctors did in those days. But a six-year-old cannot grasp that, nor can the schoolboy or the teenager in grammar school, or the undergraduate and graduate who came after him. In fact, the six-year-old had matured into his forties before he began to understand fully how the Craig-y-nos experience had affected his emotional development, his feelings and behaviour. So, what is the way to put into perspective my fourteen isolated months high in the valley of the Tawe? I finally understand that it is only *because* of Craig-y-nos that sixty years later I can sit at my computer, telling you about my experience in the hospital. The shy boy who left the place in 1947 became confident enough to speak in public in front of large audiences, and referee international football games in stadiums filled with tens of thousands of fans. The skinny kid who nearly drowned, eventually played water-polo for his university and then taught life-saving and water-safety for the Red Cross. The education he received was a sufficient foundation for him to catch up to his contemporaries and progress to university and graduate school.

He may have lost more than a year in Craig-y-nos, but he gained a life, and here, sitting in a farmhouse in the midst of walnut and fruit orchards in the central valley of California, he still breathes, as others in the ward with my sister do not. Now he sees that the granuloma still visible in his lung, scarred by the bacterial activity so long ago, is not a stigma, but a medal.

Robert is a freelance science and technology writer in California.

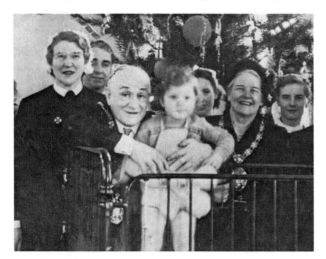

Vera standing in her cot with an (unidentified) mayor and mayoress, Christmas 1942. Matron Nona Evans stands behind the mayor. Courtesy Vera Blewett.

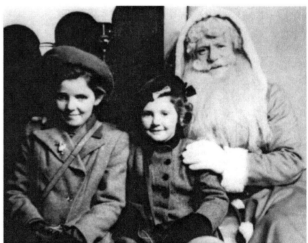

Santa Claus with Ruth (left) and Mary, the daughters of Dr Williams. Santa was played every Christmas throughout the 1940s and 1950s by Jenkyn Evans, the hospital dentist. Courtesy Mary Sutton-Coulson.

June Davies (Bevan) – The girl who wasn't there

Dr Hubbard said, 'This child's hair is too long.' I had a mass of curls. She said, 'It's got to be cut.' And they cut all my curls off. My mother went to ask why, and Dr Hubbard said, 'Because all the strength's going in the hair and not in the body.' My mother said, 'Oh.'

I remember going up to the top room, looking out of the window and waiting there for my mother to come because she was only allowed once a month to visit me. And then she'd come in with all these toys and different things, and I'd throw them all on the floor and say, 'I don't want them. No, I *don't* want them, take them home.' But my father used to cry all the time so they stopped him from coming to see me. When I was out on the veranda, the next patient to me was a shy little girl like me, and when I woke up in the morning, I put my hand to have a look for her and she wasn't there. So, I said to the nurse - Sister Morgan, she was. I said to her, 'Where's so and so?' 'Oh,' she said, 'She's had to go home for a little while because she's missing her mother.' So, I said, 'Well, I'm missing *my* mammy, too.' But she had died in the night. I was thinking then after, 'If she's gone home, why can't I go home?' I was only three.

There was no treatment for TB then. It was just fresh air and fruit and things like that. No milky foods at all, no cheese, no butter, because they thought the TB bug was coming from butter and milk. When I went to pre-nursing in a TB ward, they used to give streptomycin injections to the patients there. My TB never came back but I developed MS when I was about twenty.

June qualified as a State Registered Nurse. She has one son and two grandchildren.

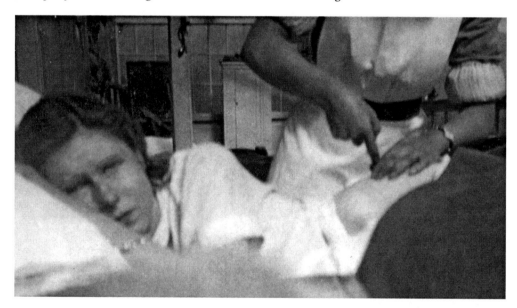

Girl receiving streptomycin injection. Streptomycin, discovered in the United States, was tested successfully on patients in Britain in 1947 and widely available by the end of the 1940s. Courtesy Christine Perry.

Margaret Thomas (Hughes Richards) – President Eisenhower's socks

They asked my mother if she wanted me at home or in hospital because I had TB in the lining of the stomach. They said there was no hope for me. She said, 'I'd rather her go to hospital. She'll listen to you in hospital, she won't listen to me.' For years I resented my mother for that, for years. It was wartime and I was nine.

I wasn't allowed out of bed at all. When they were doing the beds you would go up the top of the bed and then you would jump to the bottom of the bed. It was comical looking back over it. When we were up, say for an hour or two or longer, we were allowed to go for walks in the grounds. There were two swans on the lake, Wendy and Peter, and I remember a fox killed Peter one evening. We were all upset about it. We were very creative when I think about it because we didn't have school. We had dolls, and my mother couldn't understand why I was using so much toothpaste. We were getting the nurses to give us cardboard and making splints and winding bandages round the dolls' legs and plastering them with toothpaste to make plaster of Paris. I remember Sheila Corrigan from Barry Island had TB in the spine and she was lying in a casing made out of plaster of Paris, like in a coffin.

I had lost a lot of schooling but I've been very creative. I used to work in a sock factory, making and designing socks. I did make three pairs of socks for President Eisenhower, which had golf clubs and a ball worked into the design and the initials I.K.E. Then I trained as a hairdresser and went into my own business. I was cured of TB. Unfortunately, I couldn't have children.

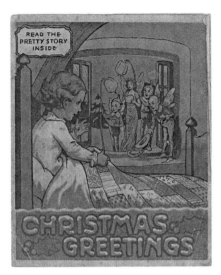

Greetings card sent to
Margaret in Craig-y-nos.
Courtesy Margaret
Thomas.

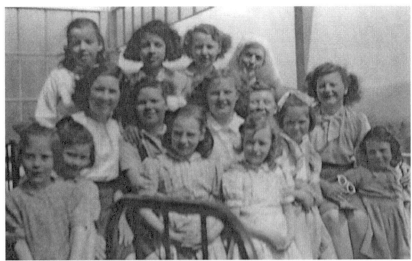

Girls on the balcony
with Sister Morgan
(back row, right).
Courtesy Mary Ireland.

Pamela Hamer (Osmond) – The night visitor

One night I had a horrendous experience. I was in bed – well, I was always in bed, I had a plaster bed - and I was out on the veranda. I could feel something in the bed and I couldn't move because I was strapped. It ran up past my legs and touched my arm. It was a rat and I was screaming. Nurse came round then and oh, she was a lovely nurse. She said, 'Listen now Pamela, stop crying.' I said, 'Oooohhhhh, a rat in my bed!!' I woke the girl up in the next bed to me. 'Listen now,' nurse was saying, 'Let me tell you. Now that little rat, his name is Joey, and he stays with us. He lives in the kitchen. We've just been feeding him and he only asked if he could come and see you. And we said, "Oh alright, she's sleeping mind, don't wake her".' She really calmed me down but she must have been scared knowing that this creature was around. She was so nice and I fell asleep. I thought, 'Oh, Joey the rat.' At that moment, he became a pet, not a vermin, in my mind.' I was eight-years-old then.

Pamela is married with two children and three grandchildren

Mary Richards (Driscoll) - A lovely time

I've got to be honest. It was lovely. There was nothing cruel up there. I had my ninth birthday in hospital. I remember my first Christmas and my ninth birthday. My father died of TB in August 1946 and I went into Craig-y-nos the following month. My one-year-old sister was there too, and I visited her every day in the Glass Conservatory (babies' ward). My ward, Ward 1, was divided into boys and girls by a screen. I had a boyfriend, Ken, who used to slip me comics under the screen.

I was kept in bed for the first three months and had my tonsils removed. We had tin bowls to wash in, and the cleaner used to throw cold wet tea leaves on the floor then polish it everyday. Dr Hubbard was nasty. I was petrified of her. She shouted at me to get my pinky curlers out of my hair, although she took us out once on the rowing boat. Another time we went to Swansea to the Grand Theatre to see Harry Secombe. During that very cold spell in 1947 some girls were moved indoors but I was kept on the balcony. My Gran asked if it was right that we should be left out there in those conditions and she was told that it was part of the treatment.

I can remember having letters from my Gran, my mother and my sister, and from everyone in my classroom. I was only there nine months. Some were there years, weren't they?

Mary became a cook in a nursing home. She is married with one child and two grandchildren.

Surely there was no conscious cruelty. The staff must have been practising the 'best practice' of 1946 and 47. If they did not explain that to me, well, that too, was what doctors did in those days.

Robert Evans (Allsopp)

Teenagers' Stories

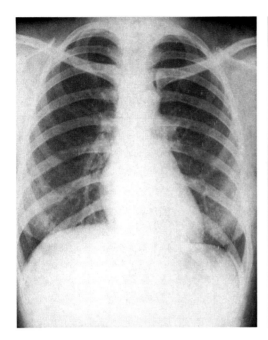

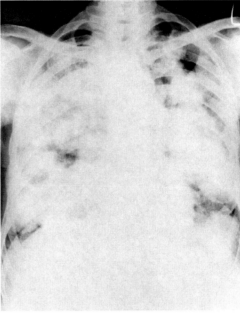

Left
Chest X-ray of normal lungs. The dark areas show the lungs filled with air. The heart is the white shape in the middle. The curve of the diaphragm muscle is below the heart. Wellcome Images, London.

Right
Chest X-ray showing severe tuberculosis of the lungs, which are filled with patches of scarred tissue and cavities filled with infectious matter (white areas). The X-ray was taken in the 1930s before there was any effective treatment for TB. Wellcome Images, London.

Megan Thomas (Phillips) – The sixpenny hop

I fell on my wrist in a dance at the sixpenny hop in Cwm Dulais (West Glamorgan) in 1941. The doctor said I had a nasty sprain and to massage it night and morning with liniment. I was in so much pain that after a month my father took me back to the doctor who immediately referred me to the TB clinic in Swansea (Grove Place) and it was put into a plaster splint. I had TB in the thumb and it was so bad that my father had to sign to have my arm amputated to the elbow. I was seventeen. In Craig-y-nos they experimented on me and saved it. I was very lucky but there's no bend in the wrist.

I was in bed for most of the time and never went out in three years. We were on the balcony from March to Christmas - in for Christmas and then out again. My mother used to say to my father, 'Joe, she'll have pneumonia out on that balcony.' We never had any heating or hot water bottles. We used to go once or twice a week for light (sun-ray) treatment. In about 1943, Dr Jarman had some vaccine from America and injected it into my thumb. They used to express it afterwards. My thumb was all black and green. I fainted once. Well, we missed our families. I remember one time listening to the radio, although it was very rare that we had a little radio on. We were all crying one night, fifteen of us. Visitors only came once a month and one little girl, Shirley, a wartime evacuee from London, never had visitors at all. She was about four. You didn't have a lot of food but I think we had enough. We never wasted it, so it couldn't have been that bad. I remember a young girl dying. They transferred her to a cot in the sister's office. We could talk to her from the door and wave to her but we couldn't go in. I think it was one Saturday night, you could see the basket coming up in the lift, and she'd passed away.

I was very, very thin - only about six stone five pounds (40.45 kgs) when I got married at twenty-one. I had a stroke at twenty-seven. They took chest X-rays and didn't say anything to me. Five years later when I was living in London and expecting my son, I had an X-ray because they thought I was having twins. By X-raying me they saw I had TB in the lungs so I had to go to Finchley (TB clinic). So, for six months I was in bed carrying my son. When he was born he had the BCG injection, and my daughter and other son also had to have them. Oh, the doctors played heck with me. They said, 'When did you have your last X-ray?' I said, 'When I was twenty-seven.' So they wrote to the hospital (in Wales) for the records. It was found that I'd had TB then. So I'd had it for five years. When I returned to Wales, I had to go back and forth to Singleton Hospital (Swansea) for about fifteen years. The doctor said, 'Look at your lungs (in the X-ray).' Well, I couldn't see my lungs for so much scarring. I said, 'Well, how bad did I have it?' He said, 'Very, very bad.' And I didn't know.

Young women's stories

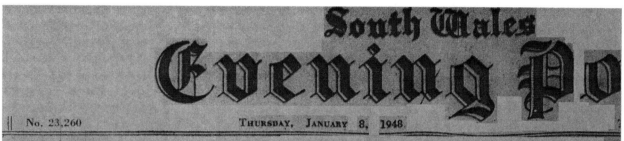

South Wales

Evening Po

No. 23,260   THURSDAY, JANUARY 8, 1948

OLE PLAN OR NOTHIN

Vales
sing

of the Irish Channel all
ft and lifeboat, the bodies
-ton Cardiff coaster Teasel,
aptain W. J. A. Jones, of
en missing since Tuesday
off the north coast of the

Weather forecast

Forecast until noon to-
morrow:
Moderate to fresh westerly
winds, backing south to
south-east later to-night and
freshening. Fair periods;
showers of rain or hail, with
snow showers on higher
ground in Wales and west
Midlands.

Bedside wedding licence bid

Bridegroom-to-be in dramatic dash to London

TWENTY-SIX-YEARS-OLD Aircraftman Gordon
Poole, of Lowestoft, who left Swansea early today to go to London to obtain a special licence from the
Archbishop of Canterbury's Registrar to marry 20-
years-old Thelma Bebell, a patient at the Craig-y-Nos
Hospital, left Paddington this afternoon without the
licence.

He is very hopeful of getting
it, however, in time to marry
before he leaves for overseas
duty next Wednesday.
A.C. Poole told the "Evening
Post" to-day that he will have
to send letters from the doctor
at the hospital approving the
marriage, from his parents and
from his fiancee's father.
When that is done, he thinks
the special licence will be
granted.
"I will not have to come to
London again before the
licence is granted," he said, "I
have paid the £25 needed for
the licence. It has been a great
financial struggle for me."
It was stated at the Vicar
General's office that A.C.
Poole's application for the
licence had been forwarded to
the Archbishop of Canterbury.

TOOK LETTER

A.C. Poole took with him to
London a letter—delivered to
him by an "Evening Post"
reporter—from the Rev. D. L.
Williams, Rector of Ystradgynlais and Surrogate in the
area for the Diocese of Swansea
and Brecon, instructing him
on how to obtain the special
licence.
He also took with him £30—
wired by his parents—to pay
for it.
The all-important letter
came as a sequel to days of
extensive inquiries by the
bridegroom-to-be, whose hopes
of the marriage taking place
before his departure next
Wednesday for a three-years
tour of duty overseas had
almost diminished.

RECTOR'S LETTER

In the letter, written by the
Rev. D. L. Williams, whom
Poole had telephoned for

Death of Richard Tauber

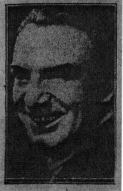

Voice that millions

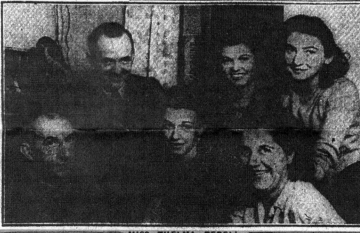

m Llandilo

errace, Llandilo, to-day, Cap-
ain Jones's young wife, Mrs.
etty Jones, and her three
mall children, still awaited
more news.
She and her husband grew

MISS THELMA BEBELL,
the 20-year-old Swansea
bride-to-be, photographed at
Craig-y-Nos hospital with a
nursing sister, is in the top
picture. Below is MR.
GORDON POOLE, the
R.A.F. bridegroom-to-be,
seen at the bride's home
with members of her family.

800 passengers in sinking Russian liner

Seven rescue ships

Betty Thomas (Dowdle) – Abortion

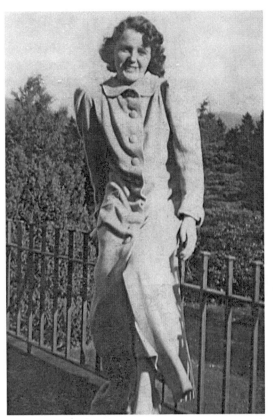

The first morning I got there, the girl in the next bed said, 'Be careful about your porridge.' There were maggots in the porridge so I left it. The Sister said, 'You eat it and put the maggots alongside'. Well, it was wartime (1941) and food was very scarce and rationed, and there were five hundred people on the waiting list for Craig-y-nos. I was flat on my back for three weeks. Once, I bent over to get something out of the locker and Sister gave me a real telling off. She said, 'If one lung is bad and presses on the good lung, the TB will spread.' But no one explained what was happening to you. The only treatment I had was fourteen gold injections.

Ward 4 (the Annexe) was divided into two, ten beds in each, with offices and rooms in between. When we had promotion, as I called it, from bed-rest and could walk to the toilet, we were not allowed to stop at anyone's bed to speak. Sometimes, a bed would be moved into a side ward and you knew someone was dying. One of the patients, Lorraine, was so ill. She used to joke, 'If they ask what you would like to eat - would you like chicken? - you know that you're on your way out.' As I passed her bed one day, she said, 'Aren't they kind here. They asked me today would I like chicken.' Of the ten people I was with for nearly seven months, I was the only one who survived. I never washed my hair in all that time. I used to put a little drop of water on it and brush it. When I went home, I had to ask permission to wash my hair at the TB clinic in Swansea, and I also asked permission to get married. You always had to have your own handkerchief. In Craig-y-nos, I wore a little white bag round my neck with number 81 on it, and 81 on my handkerchief. I had to wear it always. No handkerchiefs in pockets. It was the same in Llanybyther Sanatorium. I was number 8 there. When you were examined by a doctor you had your handkerchief out, turned your head to the side, and when they asked you to cough, it was in your handkerchief. You always had to turn your head away. I was twenty and, of course, could leave the hospital anytime but if you did, they wouldn't bother with you because you took your own discharge.

When we were allowed forty-five minute walks, the women walked along a path and round the lake. The men's walk was over the little bridge and onto an island covered with rhododendrons - and never the twain should meet. We used to go to the Patti theatre to a film show and the only time that we were aware of the children was when we passed through the rose garden at the front. You could hear them. You never saw any children, ever. The great joy was *beautiful* ice cream from the American soldiers stationed at Morriston, outside Swansea. They used to send it up twice a week.

I went into Llanybyther in April 1942, for six months, and my sister (whose daughter Gaye was born two days after I'd been admitted to Craig-y-nos) went into Craig-y-nos. It was very hard on my mother and money wasn't flowing. I couldn't work when I came out although I was quite well. No one would employ you if you said that you had TB. I chummed up with a friend and we used to go to the pictures together. One day I went for tea to her house, and I had a different cup, saucer and plate to her and her mother. Of course, nothing was said but I knew what was between us then. I got married in July 1943 and became pregnant in November 1944. I went down to the clinic for one of my check-ups, saw a doctor, and asked, 'Is it alright?' I was told, 'Fine, do you want the child?' 'Well, of course I want the child.' So I came merrily home. I went down again when I was four and a half months pregnant, and the Sister asked, 'Are you *pregnant*?' I said, 'Yes, I've seen Dr Ward.' She was horrified. 'No way can you have this child.' I asked why not, 'I shall be fine.' 'Oh, you'll have a wonderful pregnancy but if you've got a child that you've got to get up in the night to, and you get overtired, your TB will be back and who's going to look after the child then - your mother and your husband?' That's what they told me. They arranged for me to have an abortion. I was five months pregnant. My husband wasn't even consulted. He was away working in Oxford. He was never in the picture, never asked. I had this pregnancy terminated. A terrible, terrible time it was. The lady doctor said, 'You see, my dear, when an apple is ready to be picked, it'll come off in your hand but when it is not ripe, you've got to tug. They sent for my mother and she asked if I would be alright. The Sister said, 'As long as she doesn't have any infection.' It was a little boy, you know, and I thought to myself, sometimes when babies are stillborn, they have a little funeral.

Betty lives in Swansea

Thelma Poole (Bebell) – First wedding in Patti Theatre

A young girl, stricken with tuberculosis and lying in a remote Welsh castle, marries her fiancé before he leaves to fight in a war. This reads like the theme of a romantic Victorian novel but it took place on 12 January 1948 in the Adelina Patti Theatre when twenty-year-old Thelma Bebell from Swansea married RAF aircraftsman Gordon Poole, aged twenty-six.

The Archbishop of Canterbury issued a special licence to allow the wedding to take place in the Patti Theatre, and it made national headlines. Although officially confined to bed, Thelma was allowed up for the ceremony, and walked the short distance from Ward 1 to the Theatre wearing her dressing-gown, and supported by a nursing sister. The officiating priest was Reverend Walters of St Thomas's Church, Swansea, accompanied by a vicar from Brecon. This was not only the first marriage in Craig-y-nos but also then unique to the Church of Wales. Hospital staff made the couple's wedding cake and provided a buffet reception in the Theatre for their friends and relatives. Afterwards, Thelma returned to bed and Gordon went off for a three-year tour of duty to Aden. Several years were to pass before they were able to begin married life together. They moved to Germany where Gordon was stationed, and had two sons, before finally settling in Lyneham, Wiltshire. This story of passion and enduring love is still remembered fondly in the Welsh valleys. Thelma's life was cut tragically short at the age of forty-three when she died of a brain haemorrhage.

Thelma's brother, Harry, and her sister, Sonia Hixon, retain the newspaper reports of this unusual wedding.

Jean Clements (Berry) – Thou shalt not knit on Sundays

I had lost weight - was 'fading away' – and it was thought that I had TB, so I was sent to Craig-y-nos. I was nineteen and had just got married. In fact, I was suffering from shock because my father had been electrocuted. He was an electrician's mate in the local power station and was only forty-two. Dad was my life and I stopped eating.

I was admitted into the Annexe (Ward 4) with other young women. I remember Barbara Pye, a very glamorous girl with long red hair. I still have a drawing that Barbara did of my leg! However, my abiding memory of my ten weeks there is of Sister Outram. She caught me knitting on a Sunday and gave me the most terrible row. 'Sunday is God's day. You must do nothing'. I was stopped straightaway. She also forbade nails to be cut or filed, although she did allow little walks in the grounds.

Opposite page
Betty on the terrace outside the Annexe, 1942. Courtesy Betty Thomas.

This page
Thelma at the time of her wedding in Craig-y-nos, 1948. Courtesy Harry Bebell and Sonia Hixon.

Sister Outram and Dr Hubbard, figures of fear in Craig-y-nos. Courtesy Dulcie Oltersdorf.

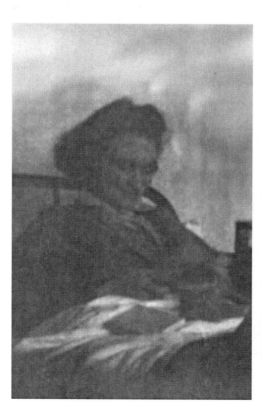
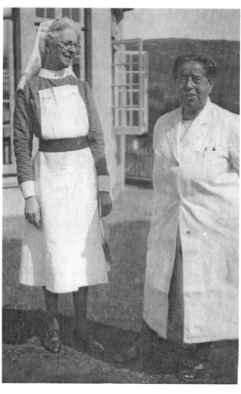

Dulcie Oltersdorf (Lewis) – Blood tests and blunt needles

I was on bed rest at home for a year, waiting for a bed in Craig-y-nos. The night before going in I wanted to go to the local dance and my mother let me. She shouldn't have, but I met my boyfriend that night, a German prisoner-of-war. He used to visit me in Craig-y-nos. I was admitted to the Annexe three days before my twenty-first birthday in 1948.

I had to lie flat on my back and do nothing. That was the treatment. Well, after three months I had an X-ray and they said, 'You will have to lie on your back for another three months, maybe six months.' I was determined that I would get better and if that was the treatment then I would do it! Sister Outram was very strict. We used to close the windows at night and she would come in first thing in the morning, fling them wide open and we would eat our breakfasts shivering with cold. It was for our own good. She told my mother that a cure depended on the ability of the patient to settle down and do what they were told. I was able to settle quickly. We had regular blood tests and we used to hate it when Dr Hubbard did them because she always used blunt needles. Afterwards, our arms would be covered in bruises. I was happy and comfortable at Craig-y-nos. It was a good hospital.

When I was discharged I married my boyfriend. We have been together now for fifty-eight years and have never had a cross word!

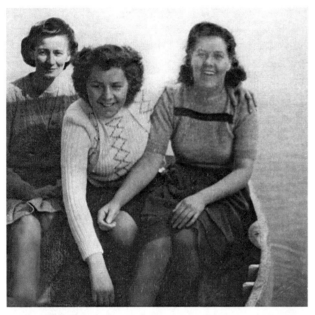
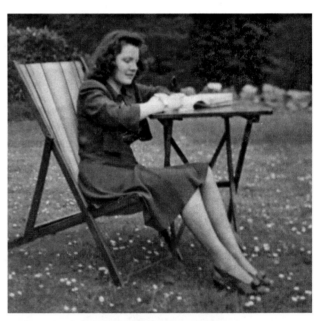
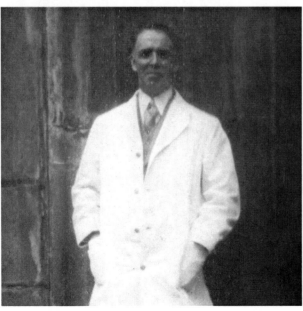
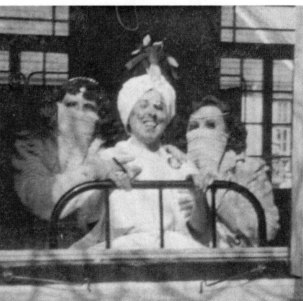

Barbara Pye (Dommett) – Mystery of the stone throwers

I left school at fourteen and worked with two hundred girls in Hodges, the gent's outfitters, making demob suits for the homecoming soldiers. It was very dusty and dirty. I was admitted to Craig-y-nos in 1948, aged eighteen, but had already spent two years at home in bed. I was very ill and put straight into a side ward. My mother was told that I would 'just fade away'. I was the only one in the ward to have streptomycin and a few of the women said, 'Well, why can't I have it?' I had injections twice a day for twelve weeks. I also had artificial pneumothorax (a procedure to collapse and 'rest' the lung). Dr Hubbard used to do it. She inserted a needle between my ribs and I was terrified. She'd give me a big slap where the incision was going, wash her hands in the corner, shake the water off and come towards me. She had a very bad limp and didn't say much.

When I was moved into Ward 4, there was an unfortunate incident, which gave me terrible nightmares for years afterwards. For nights on end, there were stones thrown into the ward through the open windows. We were all so frightened that my fiancé and the husbands of other patients stayed there all night on watch to see who it was but they never found out. We knitted, read and listened to the radio. We had earphones installed and that was absolutely marvellous. I used to cut the other women's hair but Sister Outram didn't like it at all. I was the youngest in the ward at the time and I think I was a bit too lively for her. Dr Williams was gentle and lovely. Sister Outram, standing by him, was like a sergeant major. He'd come round every week, look at my chart, look at me and say, 'How are you?' and walk on. You could see that he would have like to have said something to cheer the patients up, but in those days the sisters and matrons ruled the wards. We were allowed visitors every weekend between two and four o'clock but my parents couldn't afford to visit very often. It cost half a crown on the bus, and a week's wages were ten shillings.

I had a birthday cake, which a baker made out of ice cream. His daughter, who was my age and also called Barbara, had died of TB. You weren't allowed any food there at all unless you could feed the ward. The hospital food was terrible, terrible. Breakfast was a sort of a rubber pancake thing. When I was allowed up, I'd feed it to the swans in the lake. Some of the patients would say, 'Could you take my breakfast with you,' because we dare not send it back, oh my God no. Then we had, I think, whale meat. The swans were fed with that too. Friends sent me gifts but I never got them. I only discovered this when I got home. They would say, 'Did you have the sweets I sent up for you?' We got letters though. A little lad on the balcony, Gerald Foxwell, used to throw notes to me as I was walking in the grounds, saying, 'Oh, you look nice.' I've still got one little note here now. I wonder what happened to him. My school friend, Olive Coates, was in the ward. She sang beautifully. Even when she became very ill and was moved to a side ward she used to sing 'Samson' from Samson and Delilah - it was quite eerie. She went home and died.

I got married a couple of years after I came home but had to wait for Grove Place Clinic (Swansea) to say whether I was fit enough to have children. I was twenty-seven by then. I've got two boys and a daughter, and I'm a great-grandmother, but my first child died of leukaemia and I often wonder if it was related to having a lung tomograph (an X-ray in which a small area of tissue is X-rayed in detail from a variety of angles) in Grove Place. I did all sorts of small jobs, outdoors. I didn't want to be inside. Then my husband and I started a business of our own, producing microfilms, which was quite unusual for this part of the world. We started off in the front room.

Transmedia Data, now managed by Barbara's son, is one of the most successful small businesses in South Wales.

Opposite page

Three girls in a boat. Dulcie (centre) and friends in a rowing boat. The gardeners and groundsmen sometimes took the teenagers and young women boating on the lake. Courtesy Dulcie Oltersdorf.

Barbara writing to her fiancé. Many of the teenagers and young women had pen friends amongst theforces serving abroad. Courtesy Barbara Pye.

Eastern promise! Barbara (left) and two friends create scenes from the Arabian Nights. Courtesy Barbara Pye.

Dr Williams, the Medical Superintendent, was popular with the patients. Courtesy Sylvia Cottle.

Relatives' stories

Ruth Greenow – Mother's autograph book

I was twenty when my mother, Agnes Holden, went into Craig-y-nos in 1941. The doctor in Hay-on-Wye had been treating her for gallstones and she had TB of the spine. We lived on a farm near Glasbury, Powys, and mother had never travelled any distance except to the market in Hereford, and once to Devon and saw the sea.

We asked how long she would be in hospital and were told at least one year. We had a car so we drove to Craig-y-nos, over the Brecon Beacons. It was like a foreign country. Mother had to lie flat on her back, complete bed rest. She was in Adelina Patti's bedroom. The staff and patients would talk in Welsh and ignore her. The Matron, a tall, thin woman, was not nice to my mother, but to me she would appear to be pleasant. Mother was very unhappy though she never complained. But I could tell, and I used to hate going there. I still have my mother's autograph album from that time. An entry dated 1941, refers to World War II: 'Let's pray that this dreadful war will soon end and ask God for help for our allies to win.' Another contains a lock of brown hair carefully held in place by a pin:

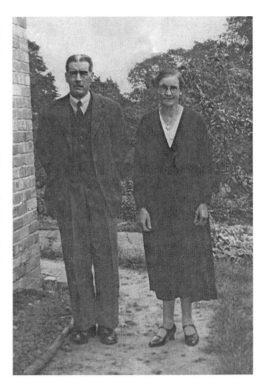

You asked me for something original
Something right out of my head,
But as I have nothing inside it
I'll give you something outside instead.
Nurse Davies

And a prophetic verse:

Now the golden sun is setting
And the earth no more be trod,
May your name in gold be written
In the autograph of God.

A speedy recovery
Joan Synnock, 11 April 1942

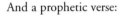

Agnes died and the undertaker brought her home, over the Brecon Beacons, in a trailer shaped like a coffin. I still feel troubled by recollections of that cold, bleak castle where my mother ended her days surrounded by people who spoke a language she didn't understand.

Above
Agnes and her husband in 1940, the year before she went into Craig-y-nos. Courtesy Ruth Greenow.

Opposite page
Dr Hubbard was fond of the small children but they were frightened of her and would sometimes cry when she spoke to them. Courtesy Ann Morris.

Staff stories

Valerie Brent (Price) – Nurses ate 4500 calories a day

I was the youngest of twelve children and lived in Abercraf, a village close to Craig-y-nos. My father died when I was a baby and my mother died when I was fifteen. I had always wanted to be a nurse so after my mother passed away, I left grammar school and Matron Knox-Thomas took me in because of my circumstances, even though I was too young. I lived at the hospital (I think my little room is still there even though the castle is now a hotel) and was paid £3.10 shillings a month plus board and keep. I had one day off a week. Nursing was in a three-shift system: 7.30 am - 4.30 pm; 1.30 pm - 8.30 pm, and 8.30 pm – 8.00 am. Because of my age, I was put to work with the very young children - between six months and nine years - in the Glass Conservatory. Although part of me was still a schoolgirl, I threw myself completely into nursing and think I appeared a bit older than my age.

I would often be left in charge of twenty or more babies and toddlers on night shifts. It was a 'skeleton' staff, but in a crisis I could call the night sister. One night, Sister Williams called for *my* help on Ward 4, a ward for teenagers and young women. She kept saying, 'I don't want you to be afraid of anything, Nurse,' but didn't explain further. She told me to put on Wellingtons, a long gown, mask and gloves then took me into a side ward where there was a young girl of sixteen. She was beautiful, like a Madonna, and I had to help lay her out. The tears were running down my face. I think Sister knew I was crying. The girl was only a year older than me. Yes, there were a lot of deaths in Craig-y-nos although not as many as people used to think. Some stand out in your mind even after all these years. I shall always remember Lorraine, a really beautiful young woman. One day she came to the Patti Theatre, very proud in her new blue suit. She died soon after, and the nurse who had looked after her had taken quite a shine to her. You weren't supposed to get emotionally involved but sometimes you just couldn't help it. She said, 'I am going to lay her out in her blue suit.' And that's what she did, instead of the usual hospital gown. There was one little girl, about three years of age, very, very blonde and quite plump. She didn't look ill at all. She had a very straight fringe and she never smiled. Quite a surly little girl, really. I was told that she was a terminal case and I did not quite believe it. They said, 'Look at her nails and feet.' Her fingers and toes were very clubbed and that's a sign of advanced TB (or other lung or heart disease). I used to bath and wash her little feet. She had such a beautiful complexion.

On one occasion I was reprimanded by Sister Williams (who, for reasons unknown was called 'Boogie') for washing negative and positive toothbrushes in the same bowl. I had no idea what she meant so she explained that some children had TB germs (positive) and some didn't (negative). Nurses had to eat 4,500 calories a day. They were very strict about that because of the nature of the disease and the fact that you were putting yourself in a vulnerable position. Before drugs came in, the main cure for TB was rest, good food and fresh air. You had to keep your immune system as healthy as possible. There were days when you thought, 'Oh gosh, I don't really want that,' but Sister Williams would say, 'No food, no ward.' Our nutrition was high, and even though it was post-war there was no rationing for staff. We had plenty of everything but we weren't allowed to touch food on the ward.

On 'Tonsil Day', the ENT surgeons - Mr Crowther and Mr Robinson - would come up from Swansea. That was a big day for our ward. They removed the tonsils because they thought that would stop infection, but they didn't know at the time that tonsils were there for a purpose (to help fight infection). Gastric lavage was a horrible, horrible procedure but you had to do it. Children as young as two years of age had 'gastrics'. Sister Powell did

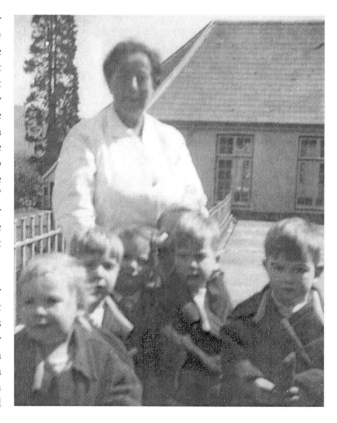

them. She was 'very firm' and one nurse would hold the child tight and put her fingers into the child's mouth to hold it open while Sister Powell pushed the tube down. You had to watch your fingers because the children would bite. Some young people would walk around the grounds for hours wearing little cardboard signs saying, 'Silence - no talking.' When I first saw them, from the Conservatory, I said, 'What on earth is that all about?' and was told that nobody should stop them to talk. It was all part of the treatment. It was to rest their lungs. Yes, children were put in restrainers during the day otherwise they would get out of bed. If nurses had time, they would untie maybe one or two children for about half an hour, but you were never allowed to leave them untied. The small children were frightened of Dr Hubbard. It was her Austrian accent and she had such a deep voice. She would walk down the stone steps into the Conservatory and say, 'Hello my little children.' She would go to each one saying, 'Hello my children.' She loved them all. I can hear her voice now. One day, Dr Hubbard took me aside and said, 'You must not stay here. You must go on and do better things.'

Visiting was only once a month, on the first weekend of the month. The children would be crazy with excitement, absolutely crazy. The six to nine-year-olds would be aware of the visiting dates and be excited for two or three days beforehand. It was like Christmas Day every month. Whatever was brought in could not go back out. Children could have personal toys but they wouldn't be allowed to take them home. There was a part of the corridor near the entrance to the Conservatory where we'd accept all these things and once they were over that line they could not go back out. We would store food gifts in the main pantry and distribute things equally around the ward. Nothing was allowed to be kept in the ward lockers, which would deter children from eating their meals, and the nurses supervised mealtimes to make sure they ate. Directly after each meal, three times a day, the 'sweetie tin' would be passed around. No feeding between meals otherwise they wouldn't eat the next one. Then it was bed pans and wash. We'd have sing songs – 'It is a happy, happy day, the sun has got his hat on'. We'd also sing if we saw the little ones crying. Some children would be taken on stretchers to a show or concert in the Patti Theatre. We always tried to make this a special occasion. We would put pretty dresses on the girls and they would all walk in a crocodile to the Theatre with their little bag of sweeties.

The Conservatory doors and windows were always open, so in cold weather relatives would come with hot water bottles under their coats. During the winter of 1947, the hospital was snowed in for two weeks, which meant that the staff went from bed to work, work to bed. I'd help fill hot water bottles for the boys on the balcony. They'd be saying, 'My hot water bottle is cold', and they would be snuggled down at the bottom of their beds like little balls of fire, when they were supposed to be up at the top having fresh air. I'd have to say, 'Come on back out!' I used to think they would smother but they never did. In the mornings it would take two nurses to lift the snow-covered tarpaulins off the bed and throw the snow over the balcony.

In the evenings at Craig-y-nos we had a big log fire in the Nurses' Home. Sister Jenkins would play the piano. She'd have us 'Marching through Georgia' every night, and some of the older nurses would say, 'Please can we go to bed now?' but she would insist on yet another song. We had no radio or entertainment so we made our own, although we had to be in bed by ten o'clock. Personal items were scarce in the post-war period so Matron insisted that we bought our toiletries on the day of pay so that we wouldn't take anything, not even a bar of soap, from the patients. We were not allowed to ask for time off. We had one day off a week and it was very rare to have a weekend off unless there was a very special reason. Then you would have to work a good ten days before having another day off. You had to accept everything you were given. Nurses were not allowed outside the hospital in their uniforms, and were not allowed to marry during training. I had to wait until I'd completed my training in 1952 before I could get married. Then I had to leave Morriston Hospital because they were still not employing married women.

Valerie's autobiography, *Life isn't all kiwi and oranges*, is published by Lifestory Services (2004), ISBN 0-9545868-7-5
www.lifestorybooks.co.uk

Alcwyn Davies – Porters' Lodge

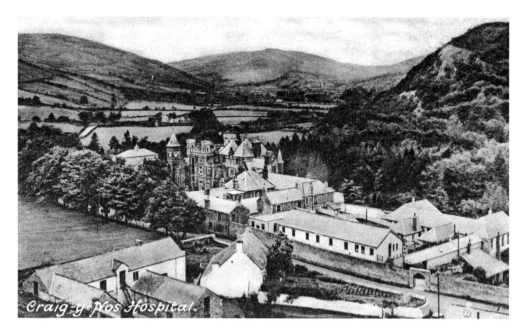

Most of the hospital buildings in this postcard of Craig-y-nos from the late 1940s were staff residences. The mortuary was situated in the square of buildings in the centre.

On my first day at Craig-y-nos, in 1942, I was sent to Mr Christie, the head porter. He picked up a stretcher and said, 'Come with me.' We went into a ward. The screens were around a bed and a nurse pulled them back. There was a young girl there, beautiful she was. 'You grab her legs,' said Mr Christie (he was always known as 'Mr Christie' - a funny chap, kept himself to himself). He seized her shoulders. 'I can't do it,' I said. I had never seen a dead body before. 'You either do it or you are out of a job.' So I took hold of her legs. She was still warm. She was about my age, sixteen.

Craig-y-nos was always a very eerie place with the wind blowing, and all those balconies with people outside, even in winter. The Porters' Lodge was on the right of the main entrance. That's where you went when you were off duty. One night, a few weeks before Christmas, there was a big 'do' in the castle and some of us missed the last bus home. Gerald and I decided to sleep the night in the Porters' Lodge, and the deputy matron, a really lovely woman, brought over a big plate of Welsh cakes left over from the party. Well, about one o'clock in the morning, there was a knock on the door and we heard this awful groaning sound. It was the chauffeur, Griff 'Canddo' (Welsh for fox because he was so crafty), blind drunk. 'You're not coming in here,' I said. Gerald and I opened up the morgue, which was opposite the Porters' Lodge, and in the dark carried Griff and laid him on a slab. We locked the door. Around five o'clock the next morning we were woken by the most terrific bellowing. 'That must be Griff,' I said. We unlocked the morgue, put on the lights and saw that there were three dead bodies on the stone slabs – and Griff, alive and groaning. He was frozen stiff so we carried him to the front gate where the six o'clock bus to Ystradgynlais could pick him up. He wasn't there when we went out at half past seven so he must have got the bus home. He was that drunk he didn't know where he was, which was just as well.

One of my jobs was to go with Griff up to Penwyllt to get coal for the hospital boiler-house. The nurses had coal fires in their quarters and sometimes there were fires in the wards too, but the only time I would go into the wards was to collect dead bodies.

Thursday was always Mr Christie's night off and I would stand in for him. He used to go to the Astoria Cinema in Ystradgynlais (they are knocking it down now). Well, I was sitting in front of my nice big fire, reading a book in the Porters' Lodge, when I got a call from Matron. 'Can you come over to the main entrance and bring a stretcher with you?' It was a bad night with the wind howling and thunder and lightning, and I didn't fancy going out one bit. As I put the phone down there was a massive thunder clap and all the lights went out. I found a torch and walked over to the main entrance where Matron was waiting. She had some candles and we went up to Ward 2. We put this chap who had just died, onto the stretcher. Matron carried one end and I the other. We went to the lift, only it wasn't working. There was no electricity in the castle. What to do? Matron said, 'You carry him. I will wait for you at the bottom of the stairs.' And she lifted him over my shoulder. It was the back stairs and very narrow, and his head must have hit against the wall. Suddenly, the man made this enormous sound, 'Uuuggh …' I dropped him and ran all the way back to the lodge and locked myself in. Matron phoned and I said, 'He's alive!' 'No, he's not.' She ordered me to go back and get him.

You would be taking out three or four bodies a week. It was very sad. Some were very young, in their early teens - twelve, thirteen and fourteen-year-olds. It was a sad, sad place but you got used to it. You had to. It was a job and jobs were hard to come by in those days. You got a bit immune to it because you saw so much. You had to. Thank God those days have gone.

Glenys Jones (Davies) – Thirty years in Craig-y-nos

I was called up for war service in 1943 and offered munitions or nursing. I opted for nursing and chose Craig-y-nos because my parents and six brothers were living on a smallholding just outside Swansea. My father wasn't at all willing for me to nurse TB patients. I had to go before a Board because he objected to me being sent to a sanatorium. He said, 'Well, if she does contract anything, you'll be responsible!' I didn't see any danger really. We were taught to be most careful. If you were speaking to a patient who was coughing, you'd turn your head a little, not to make it obvious to the patient. If a patient offered you a sweet, you took it but said that you couldn't put it in your mouth because you were busy. We were expected to abide by the rules, which we did. I don't recall any nurse working in Craig-y-nos who became a patient, but we admitted nurses from Swansea General Hospital with TB, and some had advanced disease. Three of them, I remember, died. Nurses at other hospitals were not X-rayed as frequently as we were.

When I first went to Craig-y-nos, there was gossip about it being the place you went to die, but of course there was no drug treatment then. A few children died before streptomycin but not to the extent that was believed. Sometimes, we would take people home to die. In my early days, I remember running back to the ward after lunch and Matron Evans stopped me, saying, 'Go back and walk.' I had to go back to the bottom of the stairs on Ward 2 and walk along the corridor. 'Now,' she said, 'The only time you run is for a fire or a haemoptysis.' That's when I learned what haemoptysis (lung haemorrhage) was. Years later, I was on night duty in the six-bedded ward and a little woman, who had a child about six months old, was knitting and showing me what she had done. Later, the bell rang for emergency, and hers was the first haemoptysis I ever saw. She was only in her twenties and she died. She was talking to you one minute and gone the next. Very advanced TB, of course, but it did live with me for a long time. At that time there were no internal phones in the hospital so each ward rang a bell – Ward 1 would ring the bell once, Ward 2 twice, and so on. Death was always very upsetting - really, really awful. I remember a little girl called Ann on Ward 2 who died around midnight. While this little girl was dying, her mother was also dying on Ward 4. The little girl died and of course they didn't tell the mother but she was calling out, 'Don't go now, I'm coming. You wait for mammy now, I'm coming.' And then she died too. Oh, that was terrible.

If patients were very ill we would bring them to certain parts of the ward to keep an eye on them. There was Gwyneth Davies, for example, who went on to become an anaesthetist. She had asthma very badly. One evening she was so ill that Dr Williams stayed with her for an hour and gave her an injection even though he was on his way to a dance. Dr Williams lived on the premises too. He played badminton with us, and was very down to earth off duty, but when you were on duty, he was very much the superintendent. Dr Hubbard did have a lot of good in her, despite her mannerisms. It was her speech really. She obviously wasn't a Welsh person but you could understand her. She always wore a white coat and a white blouse, with the collar turned out, and she smelled of lavender. She had a bad limp and the children used to call her, 'Drop down, carry one.' There was something loving about her but she was very strict. She'd go up and down in the lift to her room and she could see the children and she'd be shouting. Then, perhaps later that day, on her ward rounds, she'd say (in an Austrian accent), 'I saws you, I saws you had tripped.' I know that the majority of children probably didn't like her, but deep down she was good and they have a lot to thank her for. She liked colours and she loved to see the children in bright clothes. I did clash with her occasionally. Once, she wanted me to walk the children down the stairs instead of taking the lift. She didn't want them 'mollycoddled', but I was worried that some of the less able ones might have difficulty and I didn't want to be responsible for accidents so I took them in the lift. Most of the children didn't like schooling, which they had daily. The headmistress, Miss White, was strict. To get out of lessons, the girls would say to us, 'Oh, bath me tomorrow morning, Nurse.' So, of course, we would bath them in turns – it was bed baths at that time, of course – but that was short-lived because instructions came from Miss White saying, 'No bed patients to be bathed during school time.'

Auntie Maggie was an auxiliary and lived locally. She'd shop for the patients and was very kind to them. They'd ask her to buy presents for their families at birthdays and Christmas time – a big thing for them. We were sort of filling in for the parents. At visiting time, parents would come in but the smaller children would cling to us. You'd say, 'Oh, go to mam now. Mammy's here today.' They would eventually go but they'd be running back and forth. You had to encourage them because you weren't the parent and it was awkward for the parents to see their children not looking at them, no love for them. With a month between visiting they would forget their parents. I used to feel for patients who didn't have many visitors. Quite a few of the patients were comfortably off but others were very much poorer. I'd perhaps make more fuss of them than the others. I remember a little girl from Cardiff who was the daughter of a police inspector. It was the time when nylon ribbons first came out and she had two plaits with two bows at the top. She had about six or eight sets of different coloured ribbons, which we washed every day and kept in the office. Oh, everyone thought nylon ribbons were wonderful! Her parents would bring in more and, of course, we'd take the older ribbons for other children so that they were all provided with them. We used to keep toys and wash them, and if there was a child not well, you'd give them a toy. Some children would have several toys and others would have nothing so you had to even things out. With so many looking on, the children learned to share. They'd say, 'Oh, pass this for so-and-so.' They were very good like that, I must say. We did bag searches at visiting times because if a parent brought sweets in, for example, and the child was going for tonsillectomy, it could have been dangerous.

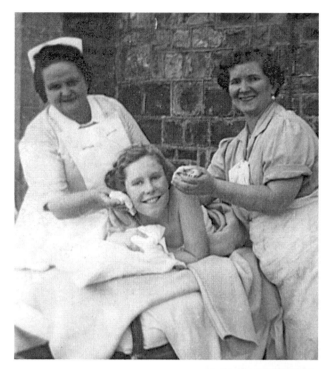

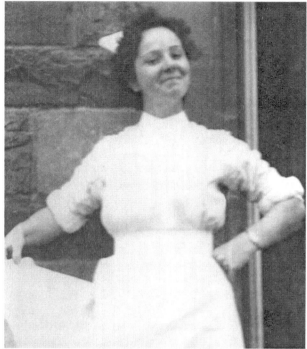

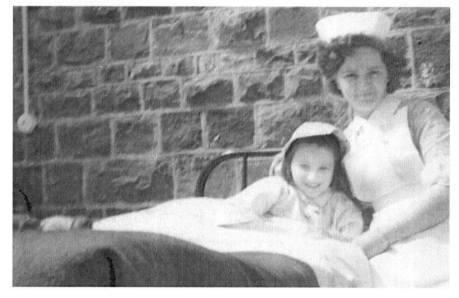

Auntie Maggie (left) and a ward maid bed bath a patient. From Auntie Maggie's personal collection.

Nurse 'Glen' in playful pose. Courtesy Mary Ireland.

Nurse 'Glen' with Ann Shaw, 1950. Courtesy Ann Shaw.

At the beginning of the day, it was bed-making, washing and bathing patients. Some of them would be having treatment such as artificial pneumothorax (collapsed lung therapy) – perhaps these would be done on Tuesdays and Thursdays. Patients who were having their lung collapsed (it was a procedure that often had to be repeated) would be taken down for X-ray screening to see whether it was collapsed sufficiently or whether it was re-inflating. Dr Hubbard did most of the APs so you'd get the trolleys laid, prepare the patients, stay with the doctors during the procedure and see that the patients were comfortable. There'd be school in the mornings for some children. Then the lunch trolleys would be brought to the ward, Sister would serve, and you'd take the meals to the patients and see that they ate their lunch. If they didn't, you'd have to tell Sister and she would go and ask why. There were patients that couldn't eat - they were small eaters - but you had to give them milk or a milk pudding afterwards. Dr Williams always insisted that the young children slept for an hour after lunch. You had to be in the ward making sure they were lying down. Some did sleep, some didn't of course, but he insisted they kept that hour for a rest. Then school would start again at two o'clock. Once school had finished, the children had their 'mad half-hour', as we used to say.

We'd only have quarter of an hour for a tea break, and during that time you had to make your bed, having stripped it when you got up in the morning. Sometimes, you'd think, 'Oh, I won't bother today,' and then you'd go over to the Nurses' Home at lunchtime and your mattress and bedclothes would be on the floor. Matron had chosen that day to check!

We only had a day off a month and two half days in a week. Patients had their lights out by 9.30 pm and nurses by 10.30 pm. The Nurses' Home was very strict. Even so, life at Craig-y-nos offered more freedom than my home on an isolated farm. You weren't allowed out in your uniform, not even across the road to the shop, which was just the front room of a nearby cottage. If you were caught in your uniform you'd get a row from Matron. Perhaps once every three months an ENT specialist from Swansea would do tonsillectomies in the operating theatre. He'd do six or eight patients in the morning. They'd be brought out from the theatre into the ante-room and the doctor would see them, and say, 'They can go back to the ward now.' Then you'd specialise them, get them to eat and drink – ice cream used to be the favourite. There were more patients with TB of the lungs than of the bones, and they'd be put to lie in various positions depending where the lung cavity was. For example, they would lie on the left side to close a cavity in the left lung. Sometimes the foot of the bed was elevated – four, eight or twelve inches, and reduced according to improvement.

Some events are very memorable. On VJ (Victory over Japan) day, there was a big bonfire on the mountainside and we all watched from the balcony. Every November we celebrated Guy Fawkes' night, and relatives, staff and local people brought fireworks. All the children would be on the balcony. Harry Secombe put on a pantomime in the Patti Theatre in 1953. The porters were very good and carried many of the children down. Different choirs used to come on a Saturday and give concerts. In the mid-1950s, a Girl Guides group was established and captained by Ina Hopkins, one of the hospital secretaries and an ex-patient. Christine Bennett, a teenager on Ward 2, was a keen Guide and the standard bearer. Sister Morgan was always worried about the clock outside the door. She'd say, 'Watch that clock, watch that clock!' Poor Christine was worked up one day and down it came, oh dear, dear. The end of the world! But it was only a clock. Staff played badminton in the Patti Theatre with people from Abercrave. There was also a tennis court in the grounds. I didn't enjoy tennis as much as badminton because the gnats used to play havoc with me!

The introduction of streptomycin was like a miracle. People whom you expected to die within days got better. At first it was given four times a day but later, we were giving it in one injection. All the patients seemed to tolerate streptomycin but after giving it for so long I had a very bad reaction. It was awful. My face would be covered with pimples. I would feel my eyes going first. Even handling the patients - just dressing and undressing them – would cause me distress. Oh yes, it was pretty drastic when it did affect you. In the end, Dr Williams said, 'We'll have to take you off the wards.' I'd been on the wards with the children ever since I started there. I was moved to the X-ray department, where they held clinics. People would come in as out-patients for check-ups. However, if I touched patients who'd recently been on strep, I'd have a reaction.

Dr Williams encouraged me to leave Craig-y-nos and take my general nursing qualification but I didn't because I was so happy there, although I knew it would improve my prospects. Friends outside used to say, 'Why don't you leave Craig-y-nos, you'll never get married.' 'I don't want to get married,' I said. The children were taken from Craig-y-nos in 1959 and the hospital was turned over to geriatrics. I left in December 1973, three months short of thirty years service, to become matron of a new residential home for the elderly, in Glynneath. Within three years I was married!

Glenys, or 'Nurse Glen' as she is affectionately remembered by ex-patients and staff alike, was loved for her kind and gentle ways and irrepressible sense of fun, as many of the reminiscences in this book testify. Many refer to her as 'the Rock', the unchanging and dependable figure in the history of Craig-y-nos as a hospital.

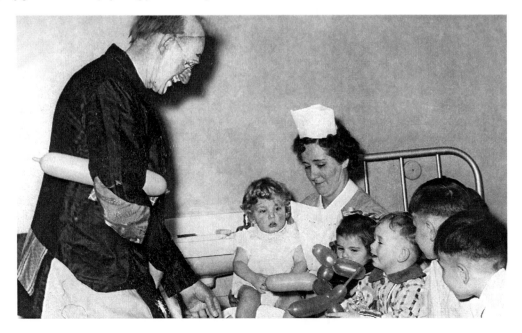

Nurse 'Glen' with the babies and a clown who makes animals out of balloons, 1959. This is one of the last pictures taken of Craig-y-nos as a sanatorium. Courtesy Glenys Jones.

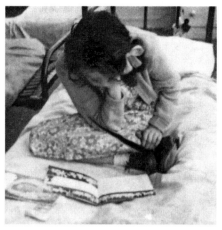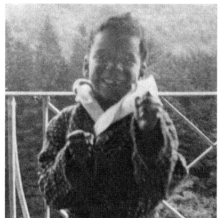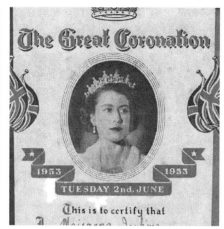

1950s

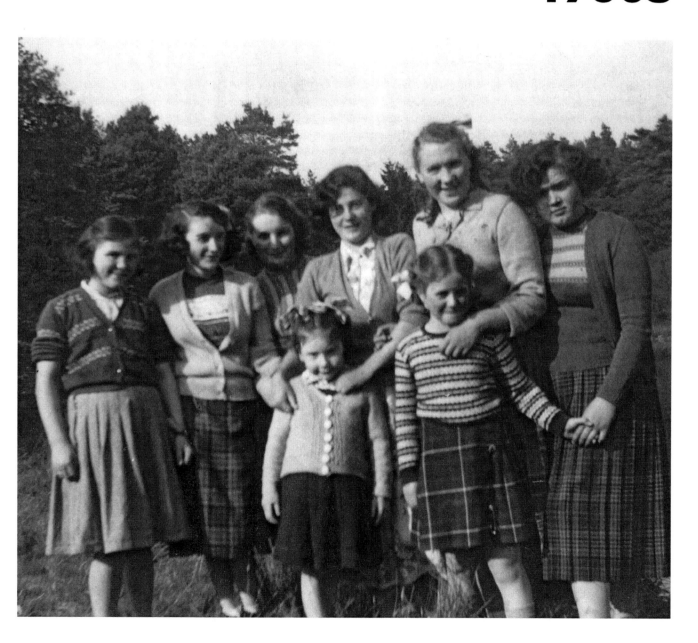

Emotional deprivation – Craig-y-nos, TB and treatment in the 1950s

By the beginning of this decade, the number of beds in Craig-y-nos had risen from 126 to 136 although for the first time in its history, waiting lists had reduced and the number of beds in daily occupancy was about 124. This trend would continue throughout the fifties due, not least, to successful drug treatment of tuberculosis, which meant that patients could remain at home whilst undergoing treatment. Nevertheless, some wards were considered to be overcrowded such as the babies' ward in the glass conservatory, which had thirty cots with little space between them and ten on the veranda. After criticism by hospital inspectors in 1945, all wards had been fitted with hand basins so that nurses could wash their hands, and the sanitary annexes were being refurbished. Sluice rooms with bedpan sterilisers were being installed, and the ward kitchens fitted with crockery sterilisers. Obviously, the inspectors who visited in October 1950 did not witness Tom the hospital cat, helping himself from the uncovered milk jug in Ward 2's kitchen! All the diagnostic and treatment areas were in one ground floor wing – X-ray and dental departments, light therapy and plaster rooms, operating theatre and out-patients clinics. Compared with the mid-1940s when only the Matron and her deputy were State Registered nurses (SRN), two more staff nurses had now been appointed. Sister Powell (babies' ward) and Sister Outram (Ward 4 annexe) were not State Registered but State Enrolled Assistant Nurses (SEAN) although they also had the nursing certificate of the Tuberculosis Association (see page 25), and decades of experience.[1] Girls aged sixteen and a half to seventeen were accepted to train for the Tuberculosis Association Certificate as nursing assistants and a number of ex-patients such as Sylvia Moore (Peckham) and Pat Davies (Cornell) returned to work at Craig-y-nos. TB institutions were quick to employ ex-patients because they understood and accepted the strict regime, were empathetic to patients and obviously had a certain immunity to the infection. There was also much reliance on orderlies such as the very popular 'Auntie' Maggie, Suzie and Edith, and ward maids such as 'Donovan' and 'Sandbrook', who were known only by their surnames. Compared with the 1940s, when day nurses worked a fifty-four-hour week and night nurses a seventy-two-hour week, weekly hours of duty were about forty-eight hours. Nevertheless, nurses only had one day off a week, or four days at the end of four weeks. Night staff worked three weeks on and one week off duty.

When school inspectors visited Craig-y-nos in 1953, there were fifty-four children aged four to sixteen being taught by three teachers, Miss Amy White (the head teacher), Mrs Thomas and Mrs Williams. There was much criticism of both the teaching and the general life of the children. They did not get dressed unless allowed 'up' for two hours or more and visiting days were only once a month, on the first weekend of each month. These arrangements were not considered conducive to successful teaching. On Monday, the 'up' girls and occasionally boys, went to a film show in the Patti theatre, which consisted of a nature film and a recreational film, the worth of which were doubted even from a recreational point of view. There appeared to be little evidence of the organised 'nature walks' supposedly on the curriculum (nobody has mentioned going on a nature walk), and the girls doing embroidery and knitting were working under bed lamps fitted only with forty-watt bulbs. Furthermore, there was not a lamp above every bed. Bedside lockers had been provided since 1946, when the lack of them had been criticised, but ward cupboards to store materials were still not allowed. The book stock was not changed often enough, there were no suitable texts to make lessons broadcast on the radio enjoyable and profitable (nobody recalls listening to schools broadcasts), and the syllabus was geared to the English language. Not enough emphasis was given to Welsh and the cultural heritage of Wales. Miss White

Previous page

Lost in books. Ann, like many of the young patients who spent months and years with little physical activity, was an avid reader. Note how close together the beds are! Courtesy Mari Friend.

Robert Spetti, a balcony boy posing as a boxer. Courtesy Sylvia Cottle.

Craig-y-nos Coronation certificate, 1953. Courtesy Mari Friend.

'Up' children (those not on bed rest) were allowed to walk in the grounds during the afternoons. By the early 1950s, boys who were 'up' were moved to Highland Moors, Llandrindod Wells. Courtesy Ann Shaw.

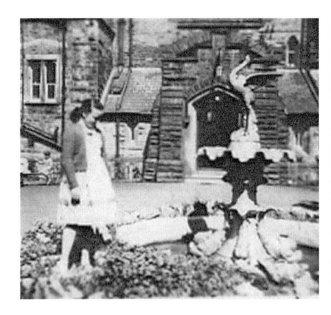
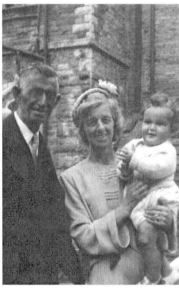

Children under sixteen were not allowed into the wards as visitors, so siblings could be separated for years. Beryl Richards' (Rowlands) sister, Wenna, waiting by the courtyard fountain while her mother visits. Courtesy Beryl Rowlands.

Mothers who were patients in Craig-y-nos were separated from their children. The parents of Peggy Jones hold her baby son, Darry, whom she could only see from a 'safe' distance. Courtesy Peggy Jones.

(who was English) was described as 'self satisfied and unimaginative'. The very young children, up to five years of age, appeared to receive very little stimulation or opportunity to develop language and social skills, as they might do at home (Mrs Williams taught this age group), and the ward sister (Sister Bessie Powell) had no time to give them individual attention. Furthermore, both the Medical Superintendent, Dr Ivor Williams, and the Matron, Miss Mary Knox-Thomas, seemed too distanced from the school's management and activities.[2] This was a very damning report but five years later, under a new head teacher, Miss Phillips, there seems to have been very little change for the better although most of the criticism was directed at the hospital practice. Only the 'up' children were dressed whereas it was, by then, common procedure in most hospitals for children confined to bed to wear frocks or jerseys. All in all, there seemed a decided lack of 'good life' for the children of Craig-y-nos. 'As usual,' concluded the inspectors, 'we were much struck by Dr Huppert's severe disciplinary manner to the children.'[3]

It is difficult to be certain where the sanatorium's responsibility for the children's welfare began and ended. Despite an apparently significant sum of money being placed into a welfare fund when the sanatorium was taken over by the NHS, certain areas seem to have been neglected or perhaps were considered the responsibility of the parents. Take clothing, for example. Some girls, perhaps due to parental poverty, had few or no 'up' clothes and relied on hand-me-downs from other girls in the ward. In two instances, girls organised a collection to buy clothing for a less fortunate child, and in the case of abandoned children, it was the older women who kitted them out by knitting and sewing. Beryl Richards (Rowlands) would ask her own mother to buy toiletries and small articles for other patients, without fully realising the financial implications of this, although she recalls being embarrassed by receiving gifts from home when other children had nothing. Ward staff made certain that confectionary and other foods brought into the hospital on visiting days were shared out among all patients but it is clear that the 'good life', as conceived by the school inspectors, was not interpreted in the same way by the hospital authorities. Perhaps the concept was too ephemeral. Whether there was any discussion between the two groups as to how the 'good life' acould be achieved in practice is not known.

In 1956, as recalled by May Bennett (Snell), Dr Hubbard announced that children would be allowed visitors every weekend rather than one weekend a month. Until then, only patients over the age of sixteen had weekly visitors. There were many reasons for this rigid policy against visiting children in hospital, which was general to hospitals throughout Britain, not merely to those confined to TB sanatoria. Nurses and doctors often held the view that children were upset by visiting and would settle more readily to ward routine if left to the control and discipline of its staff. Indeed, parents were often viewed as disruptive influences on what were tightly regulated spaces. There was also the fear that visiting might increase the risk of infection, both coming into the hospital or sanatorium and going out of it. Whilst some nurses and orderlies were tuned in to the emotional needs of the children in their care, they were themselves bound by the rules of nursing practice, which discouraged undue close contact and patient familiarity.[4] As a consequence, many children suffered the misery (usually unvoiced) of believing that they had been abandoned by their parents. This was certainly true at Craig-y-nos, where some of the very young children such as Terry Hunt, who learned only as adults that visiting had been monthly, thought that their parents had chosen not to visit. This caused problems later when the children were discharged home to discover the existence of siblings born during their absence. The sense of abandonment might be heightened by the knowledge that others in the ward really had been deserted by their parents, a not uncommon occurrence, as related by Pat Davies (Cornell). A few, like Roger Wyn Beynon, who spent five years in the castle from the age of two, could not re-establish a relationship with his mother. Lost relationships with brothers and sisters also occurred because visitors under sixteen were not allowed on the wards. Healthy siblings sometimes resented sick ones because they received 'treats', albeit only once a month, that were not available or affordable for them. Sick children resented healthy siblings because they were at home, and so it went on.

Around about this time, the child psychiatrist John Bowlby was emphasising the long-term negative effects on educational achievement, behaviour, relationships and mental health of people separated from their mothers at a young age, including those who had been admitted to a tuberculosis sanatorium (Harefield Hospital, Middlesex).[5] This work was very influential in contributing to a science of paediatrics or child-centred healthcare, and in drawing attention to the emotional needs of hospitalised children as well as their medical requirements. At the same time, a public pressure group, the National Association for the Welfare of Children in Hospital, helped to break down the outmoded and cruel traditions against visiting.

The general atmosphere in Craig-y-nos during the 1950s appears to have been more relaxed and positive than in previous decades, and this has been attributed, both by patients and staff, to drug treatment. Drug treatment gave people hope of a cure even if this was not realised in every case. Nevertheless, the death rate in children under fifteen during this decade decreased by an astonishing ninety-three per cent in England and Wales.[6] Just as significant, drug treatment eventually allowed tuberculosis to be treated at home instead of in sanatoria. One of the most important studies that helped to close sanatoria in Britain was actually done in India where doctors showed that drug treatment at home was just as effective as sanatorium treatment and, most importantly, did not spread more infection in the community.[7] By the end of the 1960s, most of the TB sanatoria and hospitals in Britain were either closed or were closing down. The story of Craig-y-nos as a tuberculosis hospital ends in 1959 when the remaining children, young women, and even the hospital school were transferred to the South Wales Sanatorium at Talgarth. It seems that the end may have been pre-empted by a confidential meeting between a Dr Culley of the Welsh Hospital Board and the District Inspector of Schools, Mr W Richards, who expressed anxiety at what was going on in the castle. In a memo, he wrote, 'I hope the transfer will soon take place as the care of children at Adelina Patti was almost frightening.'[8] For Ann Shaw who was later admitted to Sully Hospital, Cardiff, the difference between the two institutions was astonishing: 'In the weeks waiting for a place in Sully I slept with a bottle of aspirins beside my bed. I looked at them longingly each night. My world had been destroyed. Again. Should I or shouldn't I? I'm glad I didn't. Within hours of arriving in Sully my fears dissipated. The sheer dazzling brightness and warmth of the place lifted my spirits immediately. So bright was it that I found myself blinking, unable to believe it, and the view from the second floor overlooking the sea was breathtakingly beautiful. Immediately I felt better. Gone were the old sanatorium ways of treating TB with its emphasis on isolation and coldness, and visitors once a month. Instead they were replaced with drugs, warmth and weekly visitors.'

Opposite page

Edgar Davies, the head gardener, with Lady and Tosca, the ponies belonging to Dr Williams' daughters. Courtesy Christine Perry.

Gareth, aged ten, and about to leave Craig-y-nos. Courtesy Gareth Wyke.

Harry Secombe performed in 'Jack and the beanstalk' in the Patti Theatre, 1953. Courtesy Betty Jakes.

The Patti Theatre (centre) across the front courtyard. The iron gates opened onto the Medical Superintendent's garden and house. Courtesy Mari Friend.

Mary on the balcony of Ward 2 with teddy and doll. Hanging over the balcony rails is a tarpaulin, used to cover the beds during rain and snow. Courtesy Mary Slater.

Children's stories

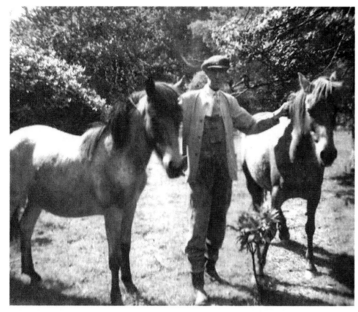

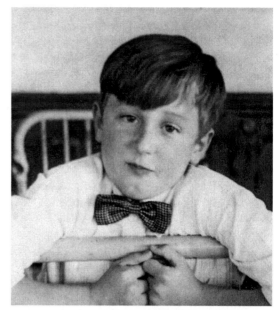

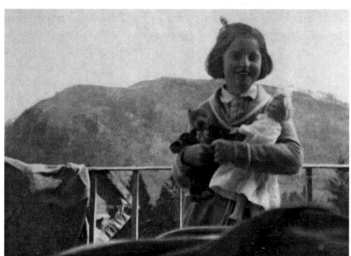

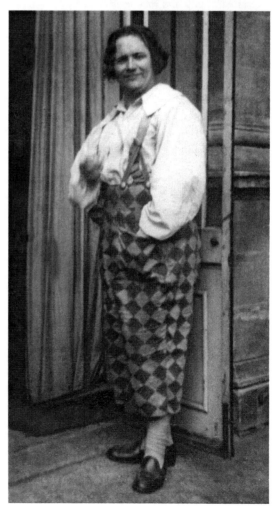

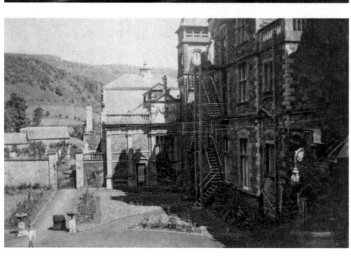

Beryl Richards (Rowlands) – Under observation

There were fifty years locked up in that one day when I returned to Craig-y-nos for the first time in January 2006 and I didn't realize that I had locked it up. When I walked into the Six-Bedder, I said, 'It's exactly the same … my bed was there. That window …' I had set somebody's hair with Amami setting lotion in a little tooth mug, and I poured the water out of the window, and it actually landed on the matron's head.

I can remember this girl coming and sitting on my bed and grabbing my finger, and I thought, 'Who is she? What does she want?' Somebody said, 'She can't speak.' That was Joan, the deaf girl. Then the nurse came and gave me a little book, and said, 'All the girls learn.' I still use sign language and I actually used it with my pupils. Theresa O'Leary, next to me, was very kind. She was much older than I was. She told me she was a Catholic and said, 'I use a rosary,' and she showed it to me. 'I do it at night for my prayers.' We were Chapel people in New Quay (West Wales) and I didn't know any Catholics. I remember looking to see if I had something, and I had an old penny. I thought that if I prayed with something in my hand, I'd go home sooner. I was always scared I'd lose it and I've still got it. Somebody said, 'What's wrong with you?' Meaning where did I have the TB. I said, 'Oh, there's nothing wrong with me. I'm here under observation.' She said, 'See that girl out on the balcony?' pointing to Christine Bennett. ''They told her she was here under observation and she's been here three years.' In order to visit me, my mother used to leave at about a quarter past seven in the morning and she wouldn't get home till about a quarter past eleven at night. Just to see me for two hours. Sometimes, my mother would persuade my sister to come with her on the bus for company. She wasn't allowed to come into the ward to see me so she stood for two hours beside the fountain on her own. She was only nine and a half.

When I first went in (1956) they gave me a little tablet called Rimifon, then they started me on streptomycin injections and PAS (para-aminosalicylic acid). I used to hate the PAS. It stayed in your mouth. I lost the last years of my childhood. I was a child and sometimes I think I would have liked to have been hugged, and they couldn't do that. The nurses were lovely. I can remember a lot of fun. I think they weren't trained for our emotional needs. I was too young to be interested in pop and rock music. I'd been brought up on Vera Lynn with my mother and her wind-up gramophone. The others used to talk about Elvis Presley and I'd never heard of him. Since that time, I've been a fan! We used to watch 'Juke Box Jury' on a Saturday night. I suddenly realised there was something known as 'teenagers'. I didn't know about teenagers. On a Sunday the girls used to buy the *News of the World.* They used to read and giggle. They'd say, 'Have you read this story?' It meant nothing to me. I was still a child.

Somebody came in and taught us embroidery and sewing – lying down flat in bed, sewing on our backs. And cane work, but it was the embroidery and the sewing I enjoyed. I still embroider, I still sew, and it was because of that time. My mother bought me this little Brownie camera and it was then I started taking all these photographs. We used to walk in the hospital grounds and I loved it. We weren't supposed to but we used to cross into the woods. Christine Bennett and I used to catch the doctor's daughters' horses, Lady and Tosca, and ride them in the woods. We used to take the girdles from our dressing gowns and make a halter. We all sat up in bed one night with our talcum powder cans, tipped them out onto our hands and blew and blew until we'd used up the cans. In the morning, I remember opening my eyes and thinking, 'My goodness, it's snowed.' The whole ward was covered in this white dust. I think we didn't have television for a week as a punishment. While I was there, they made a film about Adelina Patti with Joan Sutherland and Paul Schofield. Paul Schofield sat on my bed and gave me his autograph. My father was at sea. He used to send me flowers. People didn't have bouquets in those days. It made me feel a little bit different sometimes and I didn't like it.

My mother asked me what I missed most. I said the sea and my dog. The following weekend, she brought me a bottle of sea water and said, 'There we are, you can smell the sea.' She said, 'Go and stand by the window.' My uncle was there with the dog. I wanted to go down and touch him so my mother went down, patted the dog and came back up for me to smell her hand. She said, 'There we are. Look, I've patted him. You can hold my hand. You've patted Bruce now.' As soon as I got home, I spent the summer on the beach as I always did, and I can remember going to see Dr Thomas, the chest consultant in Aberystwyth. He said, 'Look at this suntan.' My mother said, 'Well, she loves the sea.' He said, 'She's not to swim and she's not to do *any* physical activities in school. I was never allowed to take any school games. I think I would have loved netball, tennis. I do love those things now. My mother was, I think, afraid. 'You'd better not do that because you've had TB.' I can't say I was unhappy in Craig-y-nos. I was far more unhappy when I went home. I didn't belong anywhere. My friends had moved on. Looking back, I'm trying to find reasons for it because nobody said, 'Look, these children are going to be locked away.' No one did that. They put us there to be cured, and that, I think, is what they thought they were doing.'

Beryl became deputy head of a primary school, married, and had two daughters.

Alan Morgan – A family in Craig-y-nos

In February 1954, my three sisters, Ann, Gaynor, Janice, and myself, were admitted to the hospital. My mother joined us in April and my sister Margaret died of TB meningitis in October, aged eleven months. I was the eldest, at nine. For four and a half months I was tied to the bed in an iron cot. They would take the restrainers off at night. I never cried. I just grit my teeth except on one occasion one of the nurses hit me really hard. In the mornings, nurses would come around and look at the bottoms of your feet. If they were dirty you would be walloped. We were warned that if we made a complaint about being hit then we would get it worse. At Sully Hospital (Cardiff) where I went afterwards to have part of my lung removed, the doctor offered me a radio to listen to on condition I stayed in bed. I was never tied to the bed in Sully. I remember the first visiting day in Craig-y-nos. I could see the boys stuffing themselves, eating whatever was brought in - bananas, apples, sweets galore. I couldn't understand why they were doing it. About ten minutes after the visitors had gone, a nurse came around with a big tray and everything was taken. You were not allowed to keep anything.

I only saw my mother on one occasion, when we were taken into the Patti theatre to see a show. We could wave to my mother but I was not allowed to give her a hug or a kiss. When I used to write to my mother the letters were not allowed to be sealed. If I wrote asking for *Jack and Jill* and another comic, one of them would be scrubbed out. I remember Dr Hubbard waving that stick at me and pointing it, especially if she had been told that I had been out of bed. She said, 'I will whack you with this stick', but she never did. Some people think you make up these stories but it's the truth. I was nine-years-old, I can remember what happened to us. When I was transferred to Sully it was like going from a prisoner of war camp into a holiday camp. I missed out on schooling. You felt you wanted to be on your own. You never got close to friends or made friends. I started to play football when the family was all back together again in 1957. I got married when I was twenty. My three children are grown up and I have four grandchildren. I've kept reasonably fit apart from suffering chronic bronchitis.

Alan is a retired miner

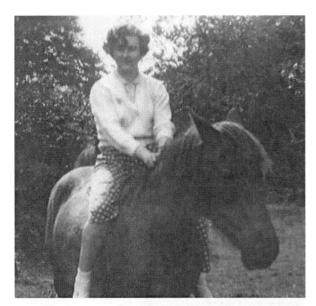

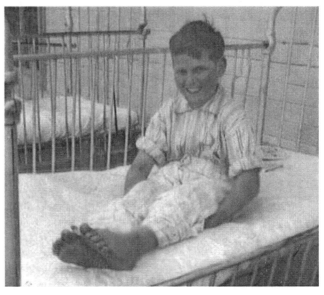

Pam Nicholls riding Lady. Girls brought up in farming communities, missed the companionship of animals. Courtesy Christine Perry.

Beryl with Tosca, one of the ponies belonging to Dr Williams' daughters. The girls used to ride the horses using their dressing gown girdles as halters. Courtesy Beryl Rowlands.

Alan, aged nine, 1954. His mother and three sisters were in Craig-y-nos together. A fourth sister died there. Courtesy Alan Morgan.

Gaynor Jones (Morgan) – Hair ribbons and fluffy slippers

I was five when I went into Craig-y-nos in 1954 for two and a half years. I had no idea what I looked like all the time I was there. We never had mirrors. I didn't know what my hair was like because that was done for us. I remember a tin of ribbons and we could choose one for our hair. One girl had fluffy slippers and I wanted to try them on. I literally put a toe on the floor and I was caught and put in restrainers. I didn't really resent it because I knew I had done wrong. Now though it would be child abuse.

I used to imitate Dr Hubbard and the nurses would put me on a chair to do it. 'You muz not do zat, you muz not do zat!' All of the nurses were stern not nasty. I realise, now I work with children that you have got to have discipline. In winter, we would have pieces of Welsh flannel to wrap our feet up. Nurses would do that for us. I was never cold. I do believe I saw Adelina Patti. It was night and I was in bed. I remember looking down over the terraced lawns and I saw three ladies in what looked like crinolines with bustles. I knew there was a ghost in the castle. I was not frightened or anything. In fact, I went to sleep. We had singsongs, not religious songs, but one song before bed would be, 'Now the day is over.' I used to see my father at visiting time. I loved raspberry ruffles and I used to eat them while he was there because if I didn't I wouldn't see them again. He was the only one left at home because my mother (two sisters and brother) were in Craig-y-nos too, but we weren't allow to see her. She was there for nine months and we never saw her. She was not allowed any contact with us except to write letters. I can't honestly say I had a bad time there and when I came home I remember crying because I wanted to go back.

My father was killed down the pit when I was thirteen. Six years later my mother died. In that respect it was not a normal childhood.

Gaynor works in a school, helping children with problems

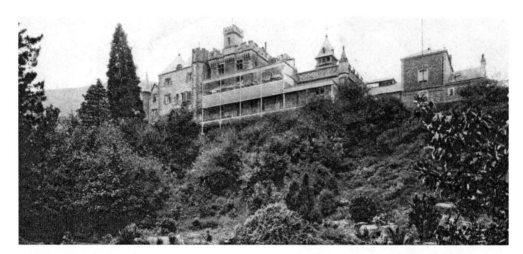

The balconies from the rockery. Some patients and staff experienced inexplicable events or impressions, both within the buildings and grounds. From a postcard, 1950s.

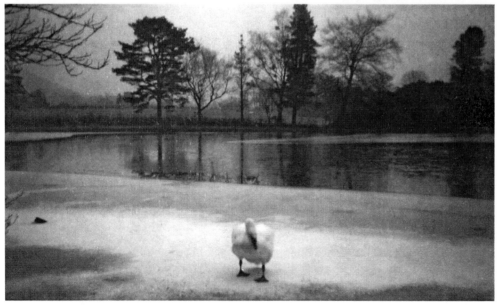

The lake in winter. It was out of bounds to unsupervised children. The older patients would sometimes feed the swans with their unwanted food. Courtesy Christine Perry.

Catherine Ann Rees (Morgan) – Too pretty to live

I was six in 1954 and I went into Craig-y-nos for one year and ten months. My sister, Gaynor, was with me in this big van, I think it was an ambulance, and I was singing 'Take me back to the Black Hills'. My brother Alan was already in and my mother was admitted too. My youngest sister Margaret died in there of TB meningitis. I remember them letting my mother out for one day to bury Margaret. The undertaker said to my mother, 'She is too pretty to live.' She had a pink bonnet on. I never had any contact with my mother. Now I think it was a rotten thing to do to children. Once we were up and going out into the grounds we could wave to her. The doctors told her she had only six weeks to live and she said, 'No way. I have got five children and I have got to live to look after them.' She told me this later.

I had injections. I was bad. I used to roll up in a ball and bite my toenails. I ripped my toe and I had a cradle over it. My sister Gaynor had pneumonia. We were in bed next to each other. She was very ill and I kept saying, 'Our Gaynor will pull through.' She said to me one day, 'Guess who came to see me last night?' 'Who?' says I. 'Adelina Patti and her ladies-in-waiting!' She remembers seeing them walking around the grounds, but she got better after that. I remember them saying I had to have my tonsils out but they took Gaynor's out by mistake. Dr Hubbard was a cruel bugger. I didn't like her at all. She used to frighten me. There was one nice nurse and I really loved her. Her name was Glenys Davies. The older girls used to take me out on the lake. A swan pecked me and I have been terrified of the water ever since.

When I got home our house was condemned but I was happy there because we were together again as a family even though we had no electricity, only paraffin lamps, cold water and ordinary tin baths and a toilet in the garden. When I was thirteen I was dragged into a car and this man abused me. I never told anyone. I did not have a normal childhood.

Jeanette Evans (Wakeham) – Putting up a fight

We made two long bus journeys from my home in Merthyr to Brecon, then across the mountains to Craig-y-nos. It was a horrible day, all overcast. I was no sooner in the ward than in came the Gospel Singers and it just made me feel worse. I felt I had been dumped there. My mother had gone and there was no-one to turn to. Later, I discovered that the nurse who admitted me had become a patient and was in the Annexe. I refused to have a gastric lavage. I was ten and put up such a big fight that the 'Enforcer', Dr Hubbard, was brought in. She was a formidable woman. She stood there and shouted while one nurse held me by sheer force and the other pushed the pipe down my throat. It was a bad experience.

I learned to do embroidery and remember being given a green canvas bag, which we all got when the teacher, Miss White – or rather Dr Hubbard – decided we were strong enough to have lessons. I remember taking the eleven-plus and failing. I also remember the excitement of going for my first walk in the grounds only to be stopped at the last minute by Sister Morgan who decided I had a temperature. For some reason I believe she took a dislike to me. I went back to my bed and cried. I was so disappointed. I never had any treatment except bed rest. It was not a happy time for me. That's why it has stuck in my mind. There was no-one to comfort you. I know some folk have said to me I should have told my mother and father about what went on but what good would that have done? It would have made my life worse.

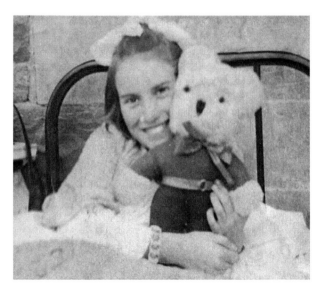

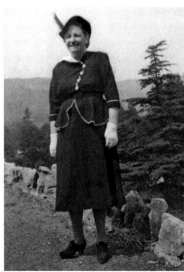

Jeanette with 'comforter'. The bear belonged to her ward mate, Mary Davies (Morris). Courtesy Jeanette Evans.

Miss White, the head teacher, dressed to kill. Courtesy Mari Friend.

Mary Davies (Morris) - A bungalow called Craig-y-nos

On Sunday 9 September 2007, I walked across the threshold of Craig-y-nos Castle for the first time since I left in 1951 as a nine-year-old. I had driven alone more than sixty miles over the mountains from my home in Rhayader, mid-Wales, for a patient/staff reunion. I had not expected it to be such an emotional experience. Ann Shaw (Rumsey) tells me I am not alone, that there is nothing to be ashamed of. Many of 'the children of Craig-y-nos' cry the first time they return to this place which played such a special part in our early childhood. It was not that I was unhappy during my time there. I was out on the balcony and made three good friends. One was called Mary Jones and one Jeanette Wakeham. The photo shows me holding a teddy bear which was a present from my family for my ninth birthday in August.

I always said that one day I would build my own bungalow and call it Craig-y-nos, and that is what I did.

Mary has been married for forty-six years and has three children and four grandchildren.

Sue Turner (Gleed) – Solitary confinement

We had to have the lights out at a certain time and my sister and I were talking. The nurse told us to be quiet. We were still talking and Dr Hubbard came in and said, 'Wheel those two children out into the corridor.' Next morning she said, 'You can put her back in the ward' to my sister, but she had me locked up in a room. I was left there - it must have been at least three days. Nobody was allowed to speak to me. They were allowed to bring food in, and they had to put it on the floor and go. I was six and that memory has stayed with me for over fifty years. My sisters, Pat, Sandra, and myself, were there from 1956 to 1957. It must have been a horrendous time for my mother because Patricia had polio as well when she was six months old.

Dad went for a job down the pit and he had to have an X-ray. That's when they found out we all, except my mother, had TB. At the start, we were all sent to different hospitals. Before that we were in isolation in Cardiff for six months. I kept falling out of bed in Craig-y-nos so they put a restrainer on me. Later, I had an X-ray and they discovered I had broken my shoulder at some point, so whether that's why I had restrainers on I don't know. I can remember the day we came home. The three of us had these stupid dresses on. They were white and pink stripes and had ruffles round the neck, like Coco the clown. Mum and Dad came to pick us up. My Dad had changed. He had been sent to Talgarth (the South Wales Sanatorium), so we had not seen him for two years. He was almost unrecognizable. I think that image will stay with me all my life. He had lost three ribs and a lung and had six months to live but I didn't know that at the time. My mother died five months after.

I'm a foster mother now. I know what these children go through during the first years of their lives and it affects them for the rest of their lives. I'm a nervous person. It came on me in later years because I never talked about what happened to us as children. The experience has affected my life, what they did to me. I have no doubt at all.

Glenys Williams (Morgan) - Isolation

Everything I know about my stay in Craig-y-nos comes from my mother who has since passed away. I was there as a toddler for two years from 1952. I remember Mam saying they used to come and see me once a month. At first they could only look at me through windows. They weren't allowed to come in when I was first diagnosed.

I don't know why they took my tonsils out. They just wrote my mother a letter and told her that they'd taken my tonsils out. They did in those days, didn't they? Mam was only eighteen when she had me so she was young herself. She had TB in 1956 but she didn't go to hospital. She was in the front room in a bed, on streptomycin and PAS (para-aminosalicylic acid). I went to the chest clinic till I was sixteen

Glenys works as a school administrator and has two daughters.

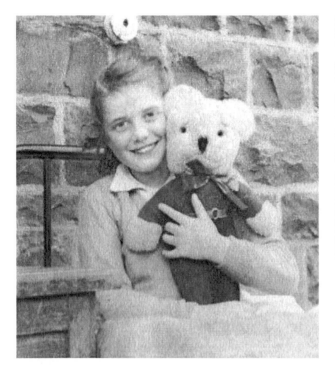

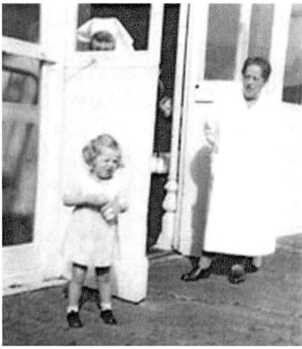

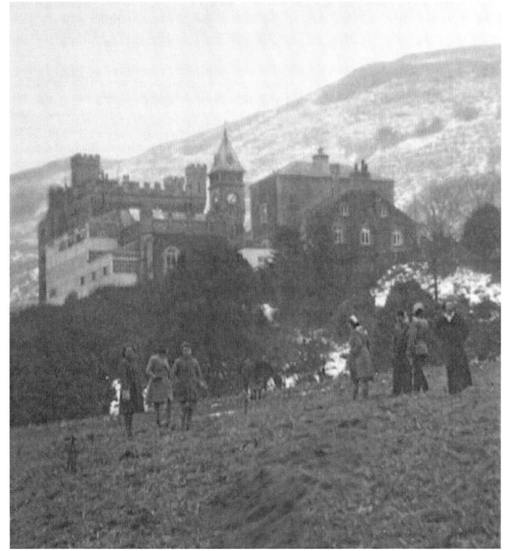

Mary with the teddy received for her ninth birthday, 1951. Courtesy Mary Morris.

Dr Hubbard eyes up a toddler outside the Glass Conservatory while Sister Powell peeps over the door. Glenys' parents would have viewed her through these windows. Courtesy Ann Shaw

Winter walk. 'Up' children were delighted to be outdoors with their friends. Solitary confinement for children already separated from their families seems to have been a particularly cruel punishment. Courtesy Christine Perry.

Vanessa Dodd – colouring the grey world of Craig-y-nos

I have no memories of being a child patient at Craig-y-nos (1953-54), only 'stories' told me by my mother through the years. I do, however, have this small photograph where I am sat in bed in complete shadow, featureless - the outline of a small head and body etched against a barred window (or bars of a cot). Outside is a blur of trees and inside, strewn on my bed, are colouring books. An enlargement of the photograph shows the face of a bewildered toddler. My mother tells me I asked for her repeatedly, but she never visited me in my gothick gloom. She was unable to, incarcerated as she was, fighting her own battle with tuberculosis in Cefn Mabley, near Cardiff. I was too young to understand such abandonment and I believe I created imaginary worlds in order to survive. At two and a half without much language, colouring the grey world of Craig-y-nos must have been achieved externally through the crayon, and internally by going inside myself. I have painted on and off during my life-time, particularly at times of social isolation, and colour is important to me aesthetically. My husband often makes references to the Otherworld I habitually retreat into, a world of the imagination where I feel safe.

Parental contact, I have recently discovered, was limited. My father made the monthly arduous journey up the Swansea valley on a milk train to get to me on time for visiting. I don't know how impressed he was by the sanatorium but he certainly was impressed with it being the former home of Adelina Patti. Any stories about my time there revolve around him 'locking up shop' (we lived in a Public House) and setting off at five in the morning. No mention was ever made of me as a child patient nor my treatment, but much was made of the 19th century celebrity, her status as an opera singer and the castle as her former home which housed her private theatre. Perhaps inspired by Patti's musical omnipresence he encouraged both my sister and I to music. In my twenties, I even spent some years in Vienna studying opera, travelling there by train (but never became an opera singer like Madame Patti). However, looking at this photograph - at this lonely child in her bed - I like to think that as Patti constructed a physical theatre in which to sing and play, I constructed an inner mental theatre in which I played and sang, spinning scenarios of my own. All my life, I have worked on and off as a musician, theatre director and scriptwriter (before moving into academia). I feel I owe my rich artistic life to Craig-y-nos and the theatre in particular, where as a theatre director I have exercised control over imaginary lives and the imaginary worlds of the stage - control denied me as a child.

Although theatre and music have always been a source of pleasure, they have also been a raft and lifeline through an early life of difficult relationships manifesting all the symptoms of detachment of Bowlby's 'attachment theory' (see page 75). My single year at Craig-y-nos shattered any chance of a close relationship with either my mother or father. I have been told I did not know who my mother was when we were reunited and I can't remember ever having a conversation with my father who was a 'quiet' man. Maybe we were too frightened to talk openly, to risk closeness and the possibility of losing one another again. The family bonded perhaps dysfunctionally, through numerous jaunts to hospitals for X-rays and appointments with chest consultants. Doctors still have high status in my mother's eyes and my childhood is littered with stories about her hospital time, the treatments she had and the friends she lost. If I ever made an enquiry about my infection, I was always told that it was 'primary' and thus minimal, requiring only bed rest. I felt my need for secure parenting was overshadowed more by my mother's illness than the shadow of my own lung. I am still told 'Forget it. It's in the past. Gone.' Gone but not gone, having left indelible marks, some good, some bad, such as the scars of a lifetime of insecure and inappropriate relationships which triggered feelings of abandonment. Although I have had two happy marriages, I remain a loner at heart and happiest in isolation, and I still do most of my writing work sat in bed with books strewn around, but with a difference. The bedroom is now sunlit, the bars lifted and the shadows less visible.

Gareth Wyke – Enid Blyton and pink petticoats

I was five when I was admitted to Craig-y-nos in 1953 and I was there until I was ten. Apparently, many children from my hometown of Talgarth (Powys) contracted bovine TB from the milk of an infected cow, which the owner then buried to hide the evidence. I was lucky in that the only part of me to be affected was my left knee. Why I was a patient for so long, I do not know. I had streptomycin. I do not remember feeling ill or being in pain before I was placed in hospital. My leg was plastered and placed in a caliper, which had a wheel similar to a cotton reel at its end, and which I used to scoot along when I was older and more rebellious. My behaviour was not good. In the early days, I was frequently tied to the bed bars by restrainers. However, my mother was told that I was very good with the babies and toddlers. I used to look after them and keep them entertained.

I remember the terrifying Dr Hubbard and the stately and gentle Dr Williams. A pretty nurse used to give me bed baths, much to my embarrassment. There was also a teacher who just seemed to sit on a bed reading Enid Blyton stories, whilst I slid under the bed whispering 'pink petticoats'. *Shadow the sheepdog* was a particular favourite. Other memories include injections in the bottom, the less frequent, but excruciating injections in the knee, lumpy porridge and tapioca, or sheep's eyes, as we used to call it. The worst times were when my parents, mostly my father, didn't come on visiting days. I used to watch expectantly when visitors came through the door and if no one came I used to hide under the bedclothes until the visitors had gone. I realized later that it was very difficult, both logistically and financially (there were five other children to feed and clothe), to get to Craig-y-Nos from Talgarth, but at the time I felt very unloved.

My time in hospital definitely affected the person I was to become. I relate to words and phrases such as 'lost childhood', 'loner', 'self reliant', 'independent' and could also add 'antisocial' (sometimes), 'unloved', and 'persecution complex'. When I arrived home I had a new sister I'd never seen before and she used to cry and say I wasn't her brother. However, despite having 'matchstick legs' and being teased by new classmates I made a full recovery, becoming a PE teacher and playing rugby until I was fifty.

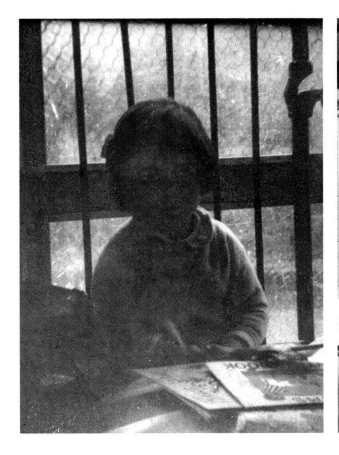
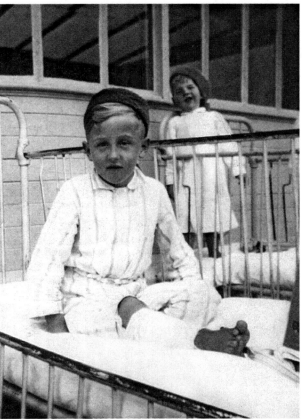

Mari Friend (Jenkins) – Dust and tea leaves

I don't remember many bad memories. I just remember the fun we had. I remember organizing midnight feasts on the roof. I was allowed up most of the time so I was able to go out into the grounds during the day too. My sister Llywella was sent home and she was in bed on blocks. She had injections every day. She was told she could never have a baby because she wasn't well enough. I only remember having one injection, with Dr Hubbard, and it frightened the life out of me. It was one where they stuck a needle in your side. I saw this big needle coming and I thought, 'Oh my god'. Yes, it was a harsh regime, but it was normal because that was the way they treated patients then. It was the other patients who helped you to settle. That's why you got so close to them because they were the ones you were in contact with all the time. They told you what was going on.

The one thing I remember about the floors was that they used to throw tea leaves over them every day to pick up all the dust. There was no playroom or day room. If you weren't on the veranda you went to visit people out there and you spent your time either in bed or talking to your next-door neighbour. The only meal I can remember was on a Wednesday when we had rabbit and mousse, which I hated, and still do. I had a doll and I've still got it. We had our own cutlery in Craig-y-nos and when I came home it was the same – cutlery, cups and towels. I do open the window every day. I was in hospital recently and it was very hot. The window would only open about four inches, 'in case people throw themselves out'. I was telling the doctors and nurses I was a child on a veranda and people didn't throw themselves out. When I had TB recently, they just told me to take these tablets every day. They don't tell you not to mix with people. You're never told to rest. It goes against everything we were told when we had it in Craig-y-nos.

When I came home they wouldn't let me go back to school till I was fourteen. I went back for a year before I finished school at fifteen. I didn't have an education really.

Mari worked in department stores in Port Talbot and London before training as a nursery nurse. She is married with a son.

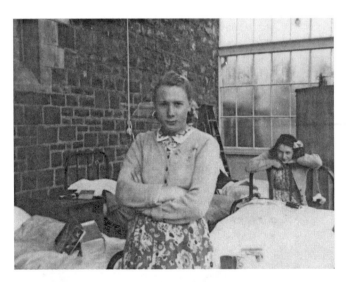

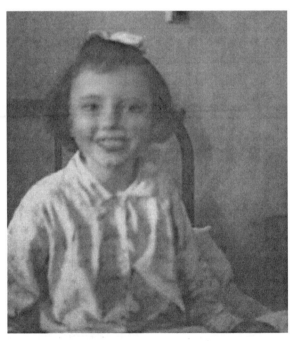

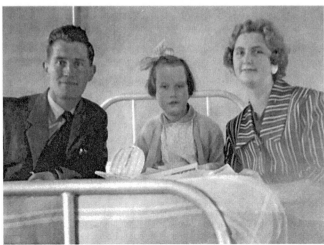

Mari on the balcony of Ward 2, with her friend, Ann Shaw, in the background. Courtesy Mari Friend.

Pamela with her uncle and aunt. She was one of the last children of Craig-y-nos, leaving in April 1959 as the hospital closed. Courtesy Pamela Bowen.

Carol, aged seven, sang with Harry Secombe. Courtesy Carole Hughes.

Carol Hughes (Davies) – 'Jingle Bells' with Harry Secombe

The Salvation Army used to play music in the grounds. We were hanging out of the windows through the bars. My mother thought it was awful having bars on the windows but then she could see why they had them. I was born with bronchiectasis and went from one hospital to another. In Sully Hospital, Cardiff, they found out I also had TB. This was 1951 when I was five. I was in Craig-y-nos for three years but had a lobectomy (removal of part of a lung) in Sully (1952). My father's two cousins died of TB, one in Craig-y-nos in 1937, so my father never came to visit.

I can remember one girl dying in the night. I wasn't more than about seven. She started coughing. When I looked I thought she'd fallen. I noticed blood on her mouth and I shouted, and an orderly came and took her out. We asked Sister Morgan the next morning, 'Where is she?' 'Oh, we've had to send her home. She was naughty.' I thought, 'Well, how naughty have you got to be?' because I got out of bed and was squeezing toothpaste all over the floor. The cleaners worked hard, and I was one of these hyperactive children, and then I'd get tied to the bed. They'd say, 'You just wait till Dr Hubbard comes.' She had a limp and she'd be shouting at us, but she was a good doctor. Many of us are alive now because of her. When I had my three children I realised we weren't naughty. We were just doing what children did. We played. We used to make flowers out of wax. The older ones used to do basketwork. I learned to knit.

Once you could get out of bed, it was lovely. Any food I didn't want I'd put in a carrier bag and and dump it. The food was terrible. I used to go down to the basement to play. There was the old kitchen there and one of the gardeners used to leave a bit of chocolate for me. We were only allowed one toy so I had my teddy bear because my grandfather bought it. In December 1953, I was on the stage in the Adelina Patti Theatre with Harry Secombe singing 'Jingle Bells'. For all it was, you were safe in Craig-y-nos. In school I was always 'the girl from the sanatorium.' I had a relapse in 1957 and was sent back to Sully. I never told anyone I had been in Craig-y-nos. I was going back and forth to Neath Chest Clinic, and when I got to be a teenager, my friends would say, 'What are you going there for?' So, I went in and said, 'I don't want to come here any more.' I explained why and they said, 'Fine, but if you get any chest problems, tell us.' Now, I've got COPD (chronic obstructive pulmonary disease). I get good days and bad days.

I was at a Craig-y-nos event recently and a woman was talking about self-healing. She said, 'As you know, we've got AIDS now and it's the same thing as TB,' meaning the stigma. I felt awful when I heard that. I looked at the building and thought, 'If I won the Lottery I'd buy that and pull it down.'

Pamela Bowen (Hill) – 'Tommy Steele' comes to visit

One of my memories is being given a children's writing set and I wrote to my father in Talgarth (the South Wales Sanatorium) and also to my mother at home. I used coloured pencils and 'play' stamps but both had my letters. I was six-years-old when I went into Craig-y-Nos from April 1958 to April 1959. Dr Hubbard told my mother I 'was dull'. My mother was very cross with her and said that I was quiet and if she talked to me I would answer her. Later, she told my mother she had made a mistake and that I had a reading age of eleven. I don't remember having much education there.

There was a boy called Gomer in a cot on the boys ward. My uncle Vivian looked a bit like Tommy Steele and when he came to visit for the first time, Gomer jumped up and shouted, 'It's Tommy Steele!' and there was uproar. My uncle was going out with one of the nurses while I was there (whilst also having a girlfriend in Aberdare!) and she kept an eye on me. She had a brother, Edgar, who was head gardener there. Sometimes mother brought my brother Robert, and a nurse would look after him in the courtyard. He would sing songs up to me and he always had an audience at the window. He had a cowboy outfit for his fourth birthday and I can remember him outside in it singing to me. I wasn't in bed all the time. I was treated with injections and drank something. My mother said I had one ribbon when I was in bed but two when I was dressed. I can remember doing exercises at the bottom of my bed because my foot had turned over, probably due to bed rest. I went back to school in September 1959. I found it difficult to sleep on my own.

I've spoken more to my parents about Craig-y-Nos in the last few weeks than in the forty-eight years before, and my father has spoken more about Talgarth. I've been researching my family history and it seems that my great grandmother, Ann Blackford from Devon, must have had TB or been a carrier.

Pamela became a teacher and has one son.

Pat Stickler (Moore) - Lamb and mint sauce

Going into Craig-y-nos was dreadful. It was my first trip in an ambulance. My mother was sick and that made me sick. I came from Caerphilly and it was a long journey by train and buses for my Gran, mother and father to visit. I was only there four months, from February to June 1950. I was never happy and felt that not speaking Welsh did not help. I had no treatment at all. One of the nurses said she didn't know why I was there. I was in the next bed to Ann Rumsey. I remember her coming in. She was the next newcomer after me, and as I was teased about the 'ghost' it was now my turn to do the teasing. But I was told she was too ill.

I was due to take the eleven-plus and Miss White, the teacher, gave me a book and said, 'If you can get through that book you will be all right.' That's the last I saw of her. On one visit, my Gran, who was a cook in the school canteen, brought me some slices of lamb and a bottle of mint sauce, and I ate it behind a comic. There was a girl from the fairground in with us. She didn't get many visitors and my mum and dad always made a point of going over to see her. Although I didn't like the place, there was sadness when I went home. I was leaving so many friends behind. I think I lost a lot of confidence.

When I was sixteen, doing my 'O'-levels, I had another bout of illness and they gave me Teramycin (an antibiotic). I was in bed for another four weeks. Since then I have developed bronchiectasis. I've never smoked but I have a beautiful smoker's cough.

Pat has two children and two grandchildren

Mary Slater (Davies) – Craig-y-nos diaries

I kept diaries whilst I was there (1950-51) and have looked at them for the first time. I had forgotten most of the events and people or, more likely, suppressed it all. I 'got' TB the day before my tenth birthday on June 17, 1950. I was told it was because I had been swimming in a river where there were cows drinking.

My diaries record a life of sending away for things, reading, getting parcels, writing to people, film shows, being kissed by boys, getting clean sheets and waiting for the weekly Long Round and monthly visits from family. I was on the balcony and remember Ann Rumsey, Joan and Mair Edwards - 'Mair, Kay, Mary and I have started the Secret Four'. I was very struck by a German girl, Gerda Grazier from Aberavon, who was there for four months and spent a lot of it playing 'March Militaire' in the main ward. I liked Dr Williams but was frightened of Dr Hubbard, and really did not like Sister Morgan who made fun of my accent, which was too English for her. When I got home it was too Welsh. I think I became institutionalized fairly quickly and stopped crying, as it was the only way to cope with it all. I can see how hard it was for my parents to keep in touch. We did not have a car and it was a two hour journey (from Brecon) by bus. They kept up a constant flow of parcels and letters. I have three sons and cannot imagine being parted from them for so long when they were small.

I took the scholarship exam in March 1951 and failed it. I was still at Brecon Grammar School when I was nineteen and it felt odd to be so much older than other people. For years I thought putting on weight was a good thing, after the once-a-week weigh-in to see if you were fat enough to go home. I was bad at games because I was not allowed to play any for a while. However, I read the whole library at Craig-y-nos, including stuff like *Forever Amber*, which was a bit advanced for a ten-year-old! This may have led, indirectly, to my English degree. Even more curious, I became an NHS manager. I have only once been back, on a really bizarre journey, when Chapter Arts Centre in Cardiff took a busload to a very avant-garde performance in Adelina's theatre. I spent most of the time remembering myself weeping bitterly over *How Green Was My Valley*.

Mary is the Wales representative to the European Women's Lobby.

Sandra Thomas (Elson) – The voice of Adelina Patti

I was amongst a group of children in the headmaster's class in Talgarth primary school (Powys) who caught TB. His wife had the disease and she had discharged herself from hospital but the headmaster contracted it. I was in Craig-y-nos as a ten-year-old for the three months before it closed as a sanatorium in 1958. We were ambulanced up to Bronllys Hospital (a TB hospital near Brecon, Powys) where I spent the next nine months.

When my parents took me into Craig-y-nos, a shopkeeper in Talgarth gave me a pink and silver tin with biscuits and sweets. Dr Hubbard took the tin from me as soon as my parents had gone and distributed it amongst all the children in the ward. It's not that I was bothered about the contents of the tin but it was as if she had taken my security away. We used to call her 'Old Mother Hubbard' - we were all scared stiff of her. I was admitted into the ward and afterwards put out on the balcony. I was confined to bed for three months, only getting into a wheelchair for X-rays. One night, when out on the balcony, we all heard quarrelling below in the gardens. When the quarrelling stopped we heard beautiful singing from a female voice. There was nothing on in the theatre that night. We told the nurses the following morning but were more or less told that we had imagined it. We were convinced that it was the ghost of Adelina Patti singing.

Sandra works for Powys Highways, Brecon. She has two children and two grandchildren.

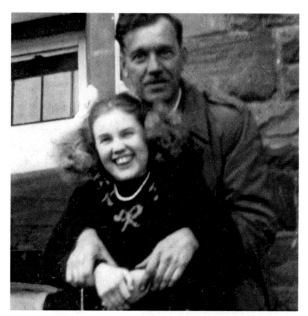

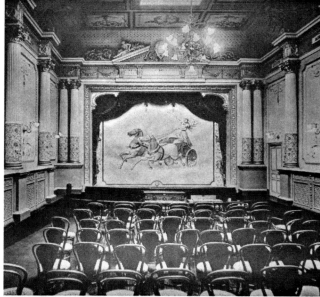

Pat with her father. Courtesy Pat Stickler.

Adelina Patti's theatre, *c.*1900. It was used by the hospital for concerts, film shows and as a badminton court for the staff. It is a Grade-1 listed building. In Craig-y-nos Castle estate brochure, 1901. Courtesy Llyfrgell Genedlaethol Cymru/ National Library of Wales.

Mary (far right) with patients and staff on the roof of Craig-y-nos. Although officially out of bounds it was an inviting place to visit. Courtesy Ann Shaw.

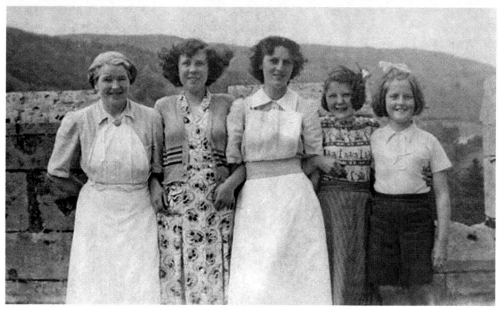

Rosemary Davies (Harley) - Made to feel special

I was not upset. I was happy to be there. I got lots of attention and lots of presents at Christmas and at visiting-time once a month. It made me feel special because, at eleven, I was the middle one of eleven children and our family lived in a smallholding in Llanstephan, near Brecon. Even the journey to Craig-y-nos was a novelty - friends took us in their car.

I have happy memories of my year there apart from encounters with Dr Hubbard who used to tear off the plaster on my neck. I had a TB gland and was never confined to bed but spent all my time out on the balcony. She would rip it off, she was a butcher! She would say, 'No pain! You feel no pain!' I cried my eyes out. I remember the pain. After that, I used to go and soak the plaster in water before having it taken off. It did not hurt so much. Dr Hubbard also ordered my long plaits to be cut off because she said they took energy away. Christmas was the only time we were ever allowed in the Glass Conservatory (babies' ward). There was a mother in Ward 1 who had two babies in the Glass Conservatory. She was not allowed to visit but could wave at them through the glass. When I met Ann Rumsey over fifty years later she reminded me that we were best friends for a year, although I don't remember her! She used to call me 'Carver'.

After leaving school I wanted to be a hairdresser but was advised against it by Dr Williams who advised a job out of doors. So I lead a country life, out in the open air working on farms. I have been lucky. I have kept well.

Rosemary has one son and works part-time in the Bridgend Inn, Llyswen.

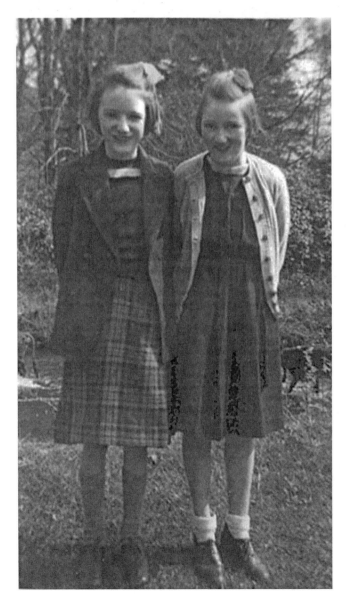

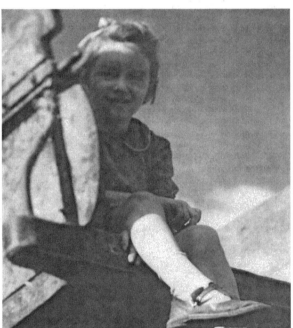

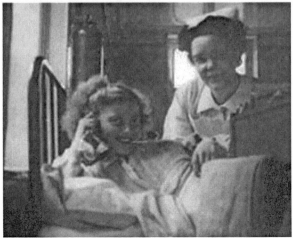

Ann Shaw (Rumsey) - Life inside Ward 2
I have changed some of the names in the following stories. The events themselves are true.

Knife-throwing at supper time

'Marion's throwing knives, Marion's throwing knives,' the girls chant. Four days into Craig-y-nos Castle and it happens. It's early evening and we wait for supper. Trays and cutlery are handed out - all with bits of coloured wool attached so that you get the same one at each mealtime. Early March, a day in which it never gets really light, and now the wind howls through the ward and out through the open French doors on to the castle balcony. Boredom hangs in the air. Dorothy my new friend, in the bed next to me, age fourteen, starts to taunt Marion in the bed opposite. Marion has a temper. She gets angry very quickly. Marion starts to shout. Dorothy goads her. Marion has her knife and fork in her hand and starts waving them about. 'I will throw them at you,' she says, 'if you don't shut up!' 'Go on,' shouts Dorothy, and Marion throws the knife across the ward. It lands on the floor. Suddenly there is a tremendous commotion and the girls start screaming. 'Marion is throwing knives! Marion is throwing knives!' Sister Morgan rushes in. 'What's going on here?' The girls start shouting again, all at the same time. Sister Morgan takes hold of Marion's bed and pulls it out. She calls for help. Other staff rush in, and those girls who are up join in too and push Marion's bed out of the ward. 'Where are you taking me?' Marion starts crying and shouting too. 'To the Box Room,' says Sister Morgan. And we never see Marion again.

Fear - Night and day

During the night the ghost of Adelina Patti, the 'White Lady' roaming the ward; stopping at the bed of the next girl to die. Dorothy says she saw her at the bottom of my bed last night. She started to walk towards me, as if to touch me … I burst out crying. 'I don't want to die.' 'She moved away again,' says Dorothy.

In the day there is a different terror. Dr Hubbard, strange man-woman creature, smells of smoke, gold teeth, cropped hair, thick stockings, walks with a limp, waves a stick about and shouts in loud foreign accent. One day she orders my supper, a cold fried egg, which I had left and cut up into small pieces, to be sent back for me to eat.

I am nine years of age, coughing up blood and very scared.

My new friend

Dorothy, in the next bed, becomes my friend and teacher. I am nine and Dorothy must be about fourteen, maybe more. It is Dorothy who explains to me that I have TB and that everyone else in the ward has it too. They don't seem bothered by it. The girls are all much older than me. It is Dorothy who tells me that I won't be in Craig-y-nos for three days as my mother has promised me. 'More likely three years,' she says. She's close - it turns out to be four years and three days. It is Dorothy who tells me that the reason my mother is fat is because she has a snake living inside her, and the reason my father is so thin is that he has a snake inside him too. I believe her, and each visiting look carefully at my parents for any sign of these strange serpent-like creatures living inside them. 'How could this be? It doesn't seem logical. Why should a snake make one person fat and another person thin?' Dorothy is unable to answer this question. It puzzles me.

Initiation rites Ward 2, 1950

After a couple of days in Ward 2, the Ward Boss demands I sing. I refuse. I don't know anything to sing. It is clear the other girls - this is an evening ritual after lights out - all know something called 'pop songs'. Having never left Ty-Llangenny farm, near Crickhowell, my remote home on the edge of the Black Mountains (except twice, to go on holiday to Aberystwyth and then to Llandrindod Wells), I have no knowledge of the outside world. All I know are nursery rhymes and hymns. Somehow I sense this is not what they expect. 'Go on sing, sing, sing!' they chant. And I remain silent.

The Ward Boss changes tactics. 'Who is your favourite film star?' Now, having failed miserably the first test, how am I going to attempt to pass the next? Other girls repeat the question. I remember the silence, the waiting expectation. What can I do? The only film I have ever seen in my life – at a special film show in Crickhowell - was set in a castle where the hero frightened people into doing what he wanted by taking his head off and putting it under his arm. No, that won't do. There must be something. Mother liked to listen to a woman singing on the radio. My brother and I always had to be quiet, real quiet, as the whole family stood in silent homage around this big brown box once a week in the farm kitchen. Is she a film star? I have no idea. 'Who is your favourite film star?' The Ward Boss repeats the question. 'Gracie Fields,' I whisper, hoping that this woman whose singing enchants my mother so much is, indeed, a film star. Some girls laugh. The Ward Boss is suspicious of my choice. 'Don't you like men?' 'Yes,' say I, wondering what this has to do with film stars. 'Most girls choose male film stars,' she adds. Dorothy guesses my ignorance. Next day she hands me a book full of pictures of film stars. 'Learn their names. I will test you tomorrow.' And that marks the start of my initiation into the culture of Ward 2.

By 1956, the rituals have grown more brutal. B (she doesn't want to give her real name) recalls that as a twelve-year-old she was terrified they would strip her naked and force her to run around the ward. She had watched it happen to another girl but she was let off by the Ward Boss on the grounds that 'She's only a child.' Phew!

Touching

One day Thomas, the black hospital cat, climbs onto my bed. He is not allowed in the ward. Somehow, he has managed to slip through the glass door. I stroke him, delighted to see a cat. I have been six months or maybe more in Craig-y-nos and miss the animals on the farm. Mother tells me about my dogs and cats that I have left behind but it is not the same. Now here is Thomas purring on my bed. He is a big, fat black cat. Sister Morgan comes in. She sees Thomas and rushes over. 'You are not to touch him!' She scolds me, picking Thomas up in her arms and hurrying out of the ward again. 'Why mustn't I touch Thomas?' I ask Dorothy. 'Because we have germs and he might catch them.' She is practical, matter-of-fact about it. The same goes for the doll, my big new doll with blonde curly hair and blue eyes, which I am allowed to keep providing she stays in her box on the mantelpiece. I can look at her but I am not to touch her. I am nine years of age.

Virgins and carnal knowledge

Dorothy likes to think herself an expert on 'how babies are made' but there are many gaps in her knowledge. Take the occasion that her pen-friend, George Williams, a corporal in the army in Germany, writes and asks her if she is a virgin. Most of the older girls have pen friends, usually soldiers, whose names and addresses have been acquired from the backs of magazines. It helps to pass the time, writing letters to these young men. Sometimes they send photographs of themselves in uniform, which we study with pride. We like seeing the letters arrive with their foreign stamps (this is when I start my stamp collection), and girls trade their stamps around the ward.

Dorothy has been in Craig-y-nos for one year, two months and six days. She has no idea what a virgin is, and it goes without saying that a virgin is a mystery to me too. We have no dictionaries to consult. Even if there was one, the girls would want to know why we wanted it and we would be laughed at especially if it was something we should be expected to know. Or rather, Dorothy would be ridiculed since I would be excused on the grounds of my age, being the youngest by far in the ward.

'You will have to ask one of the nurses,' I suggest. But there is something in George's letter that leads her to suspect that virgins have something to do with sex. Finally, she decides to ask one of the evening orderlies, a quiet gentle woman named Martha, in her late fifties, who cares for her aged mother and has a dog called Rascal. I like seeing photos of Rascal because it reminds me of home. When Martha comes on duty to fill up the hot water bottles and distribute the late night cocoa, Dorothy calls her over. 'What is it luvvie?' 'I have got something to ask you,' whispers Dorothy. Martha stands at the foot of the bed. 'It's confidential,' adds Dorothy. Martha moves up the bed. 'Closer still,' urges Dorothy. She glances around the ward to make sure

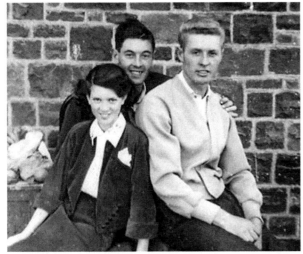

none of the other girls are listening. 'Are you a virgin?' Martha jumps, as if shot. She backs away from the bed in a hurry and it is her turn to look around the ward to see if anyone has heard the question. Obviously Martha knows. We are puzzled. 'I think I had better go and get Nurse Evans to have a word with you,' says Martha, now bright red in the face. 'Don't worry. I am only joking.' Dorothy forces a laugh.

Next day, Dorothy does some indirect questioning of the older girls. Satisfied that she now knows, though she doesn't confide this information to me, she writes back to George and says, 'I think I am a virgin.' Now, George often takes two weeks to reply to Dorothy's letters, but this time she gets a reply in a week. She shows me the letter. 'What do you mean, you think you are? Perhaps you would like me to explain exactly what a virgin is?' Dorothy writes back promptly, 'Yes please!' Another letter arrives from George. He defines a virgin as 'a woman who has not had carnal knowledge of a man.' Neither Dorothy nor I know the meaning of 'carnal'. 'You will have to ask someone,' I say. How about Miss White?' She's the teacher, a single woman in her forties, and a close friend of Dr Hubbard. Neither Dorothy nor I are considered well enough to have lessons so we have nothing to do with Miss White, except to see her in the ward every day giving out books and lessons to some of the girls. 'Ask her if she has had carnal knowledge,' I suggest. After all, it sounds official, like scientific knowledge or medical knowledge. Dorothy does not think it a good idea. Might not Miss White react in the same way to carnal knowledge as Martha did to virginity. She will tell Dr Hubbard and who knows what might happen to us? 'Look if it's something that had happened to you, you would know about it,' I argue. 'True,' says Dorothy. Finally, Dorothy writes back to George and says, 'Yes, of course I am a virgin.' Back comes George's reply, 'I am so glad. I like to teach girls everything.' After this, we never speak about virgins and carnal knowledge again.

I move on to horror comics. I am nine years of age and seven months.

The poached egg

It's strange how food can stir memories long buried. Take fried eggs. I avoid them because of an incident years ago in Craig-y-nos. But a poached egg? Well, that's different. Every time I eat one, I think of Sister Morgan and her kindness that fateful evening.

I had not been in Craig-y-nos long, perhaps a few months, certainly less than a year, when it happens. We have been given a fried egg for our supper. Food, by the time it reaches us from the hospital kitchen, is cold. This particular evening, the fried egg for my supper is not only cold but has turned an unpleasant shade of greenish-blue around the edges. I take an instant dislike to it and set about demolishing it in a technique I have perfected since my arrival in Craig-y-nos with food I don't like, which is most of it. I cut it up into small pieces then spread it around the plate, thus creating the impression that I have made some attempt to eat it. Those who are up can wrap uneaten food in paper and feed it to the swans on their next walk. Those on the balcony can stuff it down the drain, except porridge has a nasty habit of gurgling back up if it rains, which of course it does in Wales. Those on the ground floor can push it through the grating to feed the rats.

Having dissected my cold fried egg into many pieces, I need a sympathetic member of staff to take it away. Nurses I know from experience, won't, but orderlies, especially Mary, will. She takes pity on us. Also, she wants to clear away all the plates so she can finish for the evening. Mine is the last as usual. Will she or won't she? Mary takes it without a word. She has barely gone out of the ward and down the corridor when I hear the iron gates of the lift crash open. Trouble. Big trouble. Sure enough, within seconds, the loud, angry bellowing of Dr Hubbard can be heard reverberating throughout Ward 2, demanding of the hapless Mary to know whose plate she is holding and ordering her to take it back. I am in tears waiting for the return of the offending fried egg. Instead, a few minutes later, in walks Sister Morgan brandishing a plate with a warm, freshly poached egg and a piece of hot toast with some butter on it. 'Eat this!' I do. It tastes delicious. Why can't food always be like this, I wonder, trying to eat and cry at the same time. Poached eggs conjure up that memory of Sister Morgan's simple act of kindness all those years ago.

Teenage boys were popular visitors on the girls' wards. Christine with her stepbrothers. Courtesy Christine Perry.

A minor operation

Gradually the outside world drifts into the past, a dream world that we will be reminded of only with a flurry of excitement with the monthly visitors. After the first year, we cease to count up the months that we have been in Craig-y-nos with the same frenzied anxiety that we do at the beginning. We all know to the day how many years and months everyone has been in. Counting the months and years becomes something of a regular ritual to be done at night before going to sleep. How long we are likely to be in is a different matter. This is rarely discussed, for in the course of a year, perhaps only two or three will leave.

Every morning a tin bowl and lukewarm water is placed on the bed to wash. I am not considered strong enough to wash myself so a nurse does it for me. She takes my flannel and a bit of carbolic soap and wipes around my face quickly, then wrings it out in the bowl and washes it off. She will do the same for my hands. Once a week we have a bed bath, a strange procedure which I do not care for. Did we ever clean our teeth? I cannot remember ever doing so. We get occasional trips to the dentist with his bucket of pulled teeth beside him, and regular X-rays. We are taken in a wheelchair and down in the lift with its enormous iron gates, which make such a noise, then wheeled through (it feels like) endless corridors. My treatment during that first year consists of total bed rest with the bed raised on twelve inch blocks. Mine are the highest in the ward. A few other girls have their beds on blocks but these are either six or eight inches.

'You are going to have a little operation tomorrow,' says Sister Morgan one day, standing at the bottom of my bed. I am to have something called a 'phrenic' operation (see page 23), a procedure later proved worthless but a very popular method of treating TB before the arrival of drugs. Your lung is collapsed and you are made to lie on your side for several months without moving. It is thought that this, along with total rest, will cure the disease. Dorothy is unsure herself what it entails. I am wheeled into the operating theatre, conveniently next to the morgue, not that I know this at the time, and told to keep my head turned to the right. I am given an injection in my neck and told to keep still. The doctors then carry out this 'procedure', not that I remember much about it except that I am awake all the time. I don't feel any different. I am told to lie very still when I get back to the ward. I lie on my left side with a pillow tucked behind my back so that I will not accidentally turn over, and my bed remains on its twelve inch blocks. And that's how I stay for the next year.

Slug in salad

'Nurse Evans! Come and look!" I wait until the slug in my salad, a plump brown one in prime condition, gets going at a lively pace - well, lively for a slug - around the edge of my plate, before calling her over. She's busy. She's already been called to inspect five other girls' salads, with 'things' in them, which she has dismissed. 'That's nothing! You lot should not make such a fuss! If you didn't go looking for these things then you wouldn't find them.' On hearing this, one girl challenges her to eat it. Nurse Evans refuses. 'We are not allowed to touch patients' food.' Nurse Evans says she hates summer with its salads because the girls are forever searching through them, and dinner takes ages. Today, I have been going through my salad, leaf by leaf, my usual custom, and what do I find? A slug snugged up tight in the corner. I can't believe my luck. A live slug. This is a prize trophy. I poke it with my fork and it starts to move. I tear the surrounding lettuce leaf apart, mindful not to damage it, before calling for Nurse Evans. Does she not always say I am imagining things in my salads? She doesn't count green fly, even live ones, as 'foreign matter' - all part of the meal.

'Come and see what I have got!' She arrives at my bed. 'Look!' I point to the slug now displayed in splendid isolation as it makes its way around the edge of my dinner plate. It's going at a lively pace - well, lively for a slug. 'I am not eating this.' And hand her the plate. She refuses to take it. 'Leave it alone. It won't do you any harm.' 'You don't expect me to eat my dinner with a slug walking around,' I whine. But Nurse Evans has gone. She has been called to yet another bed to inspect yet more livestock in salads. She moves around the ward like a circus trainer, shouting at us to stop looking in our food. 'Then you wouldn't find these things.'

'Murder!'

Our new world, Ward 2, becomes our home, with its big, draughty windows with no curtains, and at the opposite end of the ward, the French doors perpetually open, leading on to the balcony. So, we have this constant draught blowing. There is nothing on the walls - no pictures or images on which to rest our eyes. We turn instead to our interior worlds, a world of storytelling. Stories of ghosts and 'The White Lady' are popular. Many claim to have seen this mysterious figure. They say she is supposed to stand at the bottom of the bed of girls who are dying. Once, Dorothy said she saw her at the foot of mine. I started to cry. I didn't want to die.

A favourite game during the winter is 'Trial for Murder'. Florence is always the judge, and the accused are a succession of other girls all competing for a role in the dock. Often though, the role falls to Topsy, a girl charged with multiple murders. Topsy is supposed to be very ill and not even allowed to wash herself or sit up in bed, but for the game of 'murder' she gets out of bed once the lights are out and stands in the 'witness box' - a chair behind the piano - illuminated by the faint yellow light from Craig-y-nos courtyard, and is subjected to interrogation. Often, this can last for up to two hours. Throughout the long winter months of 1951-1952, the game of 'murder' provides endless entertainment in Ward 2, and Topsy is the most popular performer. From time to time, other girls express an interest in being the judge, the one who gives out punishment, but Florence refuses to part with her role. She loves announcing the verdict: 'Guilty … execution at dawn.' And Topsy hurries back to bed.

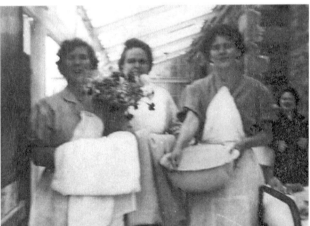

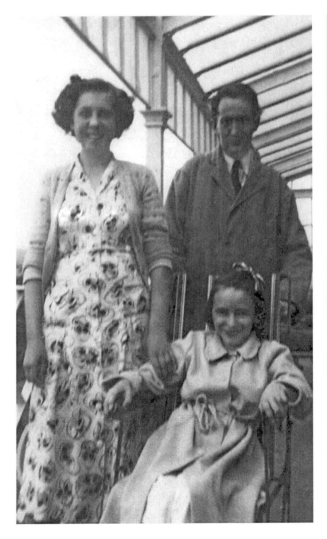

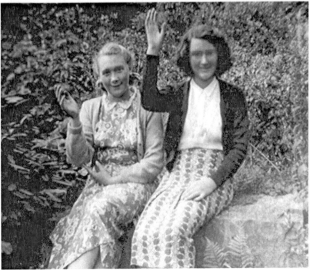

The balcony – snow girls

After months in Ward 2, I am suddenly pushed out on to the balcony. This move marks a big improvement in my life. Yet it all happens so quickly and with no warning or explanation. Does this mean that other treatments - the collapsed lung, the bed tipped up on twelve-inch blocks, the forced lying on one side - have failed? I don't know. Sister Morgan marches across to my bed one morning and announces, 'You are going on the balcony. Dr Hubbard thinks it will be good for you.' This surprises me as much as everyone else. Even Dorothy is taken aback. After all, most of the girls on the balcony are up and about. I am on total bed rest, not even allowed to wash myself. Suddenly, I am to get the 'fresh air' treatment. The foot of my bed is dismantled from its perch on twelve-inch blocks and I am wheeled outside. It seems very strange! Not only does the world now seem topsy-turvy, I feel as if I am going to slide out of the bed and over the balcony into the grounds below! I feel a sense of relief when they put the blocks under it again and the world is back to its normal - well normal for me - position.

But I like it out on the balcony. I like seeing the mountains and watching the weather change and seeing the sun rise in the morning. It reminds me of home. I enjoy my visual freedom. I have become one of the 'snow girls'. Next day, I send a letter home to mother asking her to bring me in a camera. At the next visiting, she arrives with a parcel. She lets me open it. It is a Brownie Box camera, and that starts my lifelong interest in photography. A few other girls have cameras and we like to take photographs of ourselves. (Many of these are later destroyed by my mother who does not want to be reminded of this time in my life though one album does survive, and over fifty years later it turns up in my home in Scotland. My brother found it in the bottom of a wardrobe in Wales).

On the balcony, we are a close-knit little community of eight girls, even with our own 'Balcony Boss', the girl automatically elected to this position on the grounds of seniority.

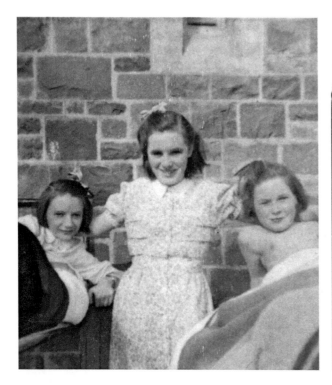

Balcony girls. Ann (left) and two friends. The foot of Ann's bed is raised on blocks and the child on the right, Joan Powell, has spinal tuberculosis and is in a plaster cast. Courtesy Ann Shaw.

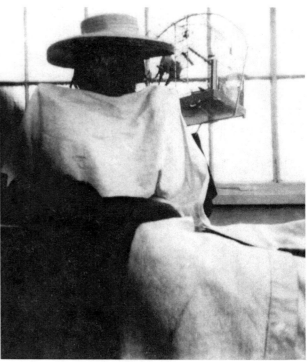

Bubble and Squeak enjoy a sunny spot on the balcony whilst Ann masquerades in straw hat, sheet, and black face mask. Dressing up was a favourite pastime. Courtesy Ann Shaw.

My father was killed down the
pit when I was thirteen.

Six years later my mother died.

In that respect it was not
a normal childhood.

Gaynor Jones (Morgan)

Bubble and Squeak

Winter of 1950 and I am brought back into Ward 2 from the balcony. It's my first Christmas in Craig-y-nos and mother walks in with a birdcage containing two budgies, one male and blue, and the other female and green. I burst out crying. 'You can't bring them in here!' I say. 'I shall get the most awful row from Sister Morgan and Dr Hubbard. Take them away. Quick, before they see them!' Mother shakes her head. 'No, it's all right, you can have them.' I stare at the birds. What can it mean? Living things are unheard of in the ward. We are not allowed to touch living things lest they catch something from us.

That first winter in Ward 2 is difficult. I am already having rows from Sister Morgan and Dr Hubbard because I am not doing what they tell me. I have been brought in from the balcony for the winter, away from my friends, and placed in this huge, cold ward with older girls. No longer is there anyone close to talk to, no one to confide in. The blocks have been removed from my bed and I am told to sit up, except I don't want to sit up because it makes me feel dizzy. Dr Hubbard tries to make me do exercises. She waves her arms around in a circular fashion. 'Pretend you are riding a bicycle! You must do it six times a day. You must do this!' I watch fascinated as this most unlikely woman pretends to be riding a bike, only with her arms. 'What for?' I think but dare not ask. Sister Morgan takes to scolding me because I refuse to sit up in bed. I keep sliding down under the bedclothes with my books. It's winter and I am cold. Why don't they leave me alone? I have retreated totally into my interior world of books, and I can't be bothered to sit up in bed. Mother, I learn later, refuses to accept that I have lost the will to live and persuades Dr Hubbard to let her bring in two birds to see if they will revive my interest in life. Dr Hubbard names them Bubble and Squeak. Those birds mark a turning point for me in Craig-y-nos. Somehow, those little birds with their bright colours, chirping away daily, give me an interest again, and I adapt to life in Craig-y-nos, to the institutional way of living. I learn to survive, thanks to Bubble and Squeak. I am ten years of age. I start to send home urgent letters asking mother to bring me in books on budgies, and even magazines devoted to them, since Miss White has nothing on the subject in her library.

Years later, I have only been home a couple of months when I receive a letter saying that Bubble and Squeak have flown away. Someone had forgotten to put the latch back on their cage after cleaning it and they were seen for a short time flying amongst the trees. After that - nothing.

Creepy-crawlies

Roy Harry says his mother was amazed when he returned home in 1946 after a long spell in Craig-y-nos, 'Singing in Welsh with nits in my hair! I was reminded of this story while transcribing an account of eleven-year-old Beryl Richards' early days in Craig-y-nos. She asked why one new girl had her head swathed in towels and was told it was because she had 'creepy crawlies' in her hair. It resurrected a long buried, shameful memory from that summer of 1951, when Frances, the girl in the next bed to me on the balcony, and I, discover we have head lice. We know about new girls having their heads searched on arrival and how they have to have their hair covered in evil-smelling liquid, and how girls stare at them. But we have been in for years, and in bed. How come we got nits? We do not, for a second, consider telling the staff because we will have to suffer the humiliation of having our heads disinfected. We come up with a plan.

It is summer with long light evenings. After night sister has made her evening tour, we get out mirrors and combs and catch the nits. We line them up in neat rows, kill them and count them. That first night produces a lucrative haul of nearly a hundred nits. We compare our night's work. I have more nits than Frances. By the end of the week our hard work shows. We are down to eggs. We carefully crack them with our finger nails to make certain they will not hatch. At last, we declare our heads clean, and nobody knows about it.

Many have commented on the fact that Craig-y-nos taught us to be self-reliant, independent. You have to sort things out for yourselves because nobody else is going to do it for you. Frances and I are eleven years of age.

Education in Craig-y-nos

Those who are judged well enough receive lessons from Miss White, a plump woman of indeterminate age. She is a close friend of Dr Hubbard. They have tea together every day and we think Miss White carries tales to her. How else would Dr Hubbard know so much about us? Miss White always wears a deep blue blazer with shiny buttons, thick stockings and a warm tweed skirt. That's her summer outfit. When the weather gets cold, she puts lots of clothes on because she has to stand for hours in Ward 2. Usually, she stands at the French doors so she can see what we are doing on the balcony and at the same time watch what is going on in the ward. Every Wednesday afternoon at three o'clock, we have our weekly service and sermon given by Miss White, and once a month it's given by a proper parson. Sometimes, we get it more often if there happens to be a parson passing through. It is good for our souls. Thursday afternoons we have singing lessons because singing is good for our lungs. On Monday afternoons we go to the cinema held in the Adelina Patti theatre 'to broaden our minds'. When Dr Hubbard decides you are strong enough for lessons, she informs Miss White who then comes along with a green canvas bag, a pencil, a biro, three notebooks, and textbooks on English grammar, arithmetic, history and geography. Scripture and hygiene are considered to be the two most important subjects and we are given a morning session on each during the week. These are the only subjects in which we are all taught together.

Miss White takes a dislike to me because she says I do not make an effort to learn. In fact, I have been in Craig-y-nos for more than a year before Dr Hubbard decides I am 'strong enough' to take Miss White's tuition. She need not have bothered. Miss White comes over to my bed one Monday morning bearing an extra canvas bag, and I know what is up. I don't know whether to be annoyed or pleased. I prefer to read my own books. 'Dr Hubbard tells me you are now well enough to have some lessons,' says Miss White. I say nothing. I am in the middle of *Kidnapped* and have got to an exciting section. I don't want to be bothered with sums. No matter. Dr Hubbard has decreed lessons, so lessons it is to be. Miss White's first job is to find out what level of education I have reached so that she can give me the required standard textbooks. There follows an irritating morning in which she asks me to do all kinds of simple sums, followed by a test of English grammar of which I have no idea what she is talking about, and some simple geography questions about a world I know nothing of. At the end, she comes to the conclusion I have no standard of education. So she gives me some basic textbooks, which I look at, decide are boring and go back to reading *Kidnapped*. Miss White is not pleased.

Breaking into the library

Miss White has a library and once we are allowed up we can visit it one afternoon a week between three and four o'clock to borrow one book. My best friend Carver (I still don't know why she had this name because her real name was Rosemary), and I, decide that one book a week is not enough. So, we come up with a plan to break into the school library, a basement room with bars across the window. 'See those bars on the window?' says Carver one day. 'I reckon we can squeeze through.' The window is permanently open like all windows at Craig-y-nos. Others want into the library too. So, one afternoon we try it. I am the first through, being the thinnest. Carver follows. Valerie, the 'Balcony Boss' takes charge. 'Get the door open to let us in!' We fumble with the yale lock, not having seen one before. It swings open and the rest of the balcony girls swarm in. So, once a week, we slip through the barred windows to pinch books (we always returned them). Miss White never finds out. One day, Carver puts on two pounds and get stuck. She refuses to go through the window again so it's left to me to break in. But Carver agrees to stand on guard duty.

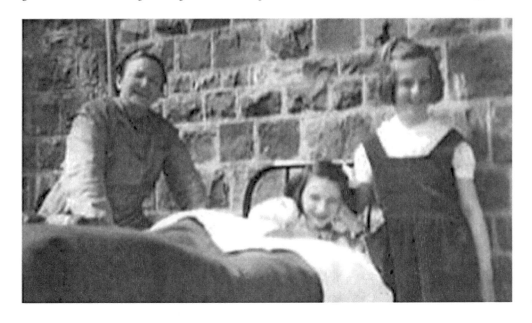

Miss White trying to persuade Ann and Mary of the benefits of education. Courtesy Ann Shaw.

The asthma attack

A new girl called Gwyneth has been put on the balcony. She is a distant relative of mine, so they tell me, and she too comes from a farm. She is older than us – fourteen, going on fifteen, and is very clever. She wants to be a doctor when she grows up. Nobody laughs at her when she says this. But Gwyneth has asthma, and Dr Hubbard thinks that putting her out on the balcony in midwinter will help. Gwyneth is given a hand bell to ring if she feels an attack coming on. Well, we are going through a bad spell with dense fogs and lots of damp air around - after all it is mid-January - and the first night out on the balcony brings on an asthma attack. It's frightening to watch. We have never seen one before and we are scared. Gwyneth rings her bell. Nothing happens. So, we take it and ring it. Still nothing. 'Look we have got to do something,' says Carver. We are just standing there, petrified, watching Gwyneth fighting to breathe. 'Let's find Night Sister.' We search the kitchen and staff quarters for help.

Our shouts eventually produce Night Sister, the only one on duty for the whole hospital. 'What is it? What is all the fuss about?' She follows us out on to the balcony. Gwyneth looks as if she is about to die any minute. We watch terrified. 'Oh, my goodness!' Sister is shocked too and rushes back to the office, and returns with an inhaler. This seems to help Gwyneth. 'Where is Louise?' We shake our heads. Eventually, Louise, the night orderly, appears, smelling strongly of smoke and squinting the way the way you do when suddenly confronted by bright lights, for by now the whole ward is awake with the commotion on the balcony. 'Perhaps Gwyneth will be moved back indoors,' says Carver. We stand by ready to help move her bed. After all, the fog has got even worse. But no, Sister leaves her there. Undeterred by this episode, Dr Hubbard orders Gwyneth to be left on the balcony for another three more days during which she suffers more attacks. It's Sister Morgan who finally wheels Gwyneth back into Ward 2.

Second Christmas in Craig-y-nos – the tropical fish

The Friends of Craig-y-nos ask Dr Hubbard what they can give us for Christmas. She suggests a tropical aquarium. Its arrival causes great excitement. It's Carver who spots a certain irony. 'These fish are a lot warmer than us,' she says, peering into the tankful of brightly coloured fish. 'They have got to live at sixty degrees Fahrenheit or they will die,' explains Miss White, our teacher. Dr Hubbard is devoted to the fish. She is forever standing at the tank admiring it, and dropping bits of food into it. She has hit on the idea that having some living things in the ward might help us (this is the Christmas after I got my budgies). The fishes' names are pinned up against the side of the tank. Miss White says this is to help our education, to learn about the outside world. Except … tragedy has struck. Louise, the night orderly, has switched the aquarium off. 'Waste of electricity,' she says. After all, none of us have any form of heating so it doesn't make sense for the fish. Well, that is Louise's thinking. It is Carver who spots the catastrophe. 'Come and see this!' she shouts. We scramble out of bed and rush to the tank. There, floating on the surface, are seven dead fish. The enormity of the event causes panic in the ward. 'What will Dr Hubbard say?' 'She will say we did it on purpose!' To our surprise Sister Morgan is unconcerned. She didn't like the aquarium in the first place, maybe because it is Dr Hubbard's idea, and also it meant she has had to squeeze the beds even closer in order to make room for it. 'I will go and get a plate,' she says. She returns a few minutes later with one of our dinner plates and a large serving spoon. Meticulously, she lifts the dead fish out and places them around the plate. 'This will be a special treat for Tom-Puss,' she says. We watch fascinated as she lays the fish out in a neat circle around the edge of the plate.

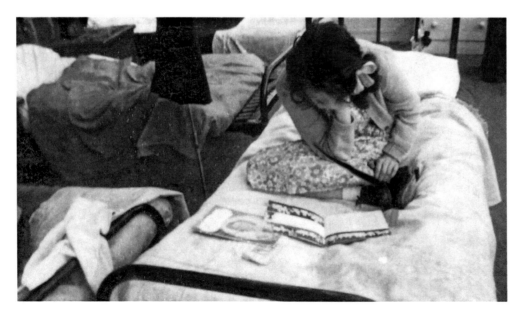

Lost in books. Ann, like many of the young patients who spent months and years with little physical activity, was an avid reader. Note how close together the beds are! Courtesy Mari Friend.

At the next Long Round Dr Hubbard stops at the aquarium. She always spends more time looking into the tank than at the girls in the bed. 'How are my little fish doing,' she murmurs, with something approaching affection in her voice. Sister Morgan tries to hurry her on but Dr Hubbard senses something amiss. 'Vot haz happened to ze Angel fish?' Her eyes, hawk like, scan the tank. Sister Morgan turns her head sideways and winks at us with her left eye. 'I can't see ze big black striped fish either, or ze red one? Vot haz gone wrong?' Dr Williams stands silently, waiting for the inevitable explosion as these two powerful women collide, yet again. The Long Round halts. Missing fish is top of the agenda. 'I thought I saw them there this morning,' lies Sister Morgan. Carver and I giggle as we sit around the big table in the centre of the ward. Dr Hubbard demands explanations. 'Who in zis ward haz been tampering with ze tank?' She looks straight in the direction of Carver and me. We shake our heads. Suddenly, Sister Morgan changes her story. 'How silly of me! I quite forgot to tell you but the heater was accidentally switched off the other day by one of the night staff. I do recall her saying something about a few fish dying.' Dr Hubbard explodes and demands to know the name of the culprit. Sister Morgan hands over the name, like a scalp, for she never did care for Louise. 'I will see her tonight,' says Dr Hubbard. God help Louise.

The hot water bottles

Great excitement! It's started to snow. We love the snow on the balcony, we love to build tents over our beds with old bits of green tarpaulin and watch the thermometer plunge. It hangs over the railings at the end of the balcony and we consult it several times a day. It's now dropped below zero - in the day. Carver and I study it like hawks. We know that once it sinks too much below freezing there is a chance that we might be brought indoors. It is snowing hard. So far, it only covers the foot of my bed. Yes, it's cold but the snow is exciting. Sister Morgan even hands out an extra tattered old blanket. Carver inspects hers. 'She need not have bothered. Look at all these holes! It wouldn't keep a flea warm.' She counts the holes. 'That's what it *has* been keeping warm,' say I, not showing much sympathy. My blanket has fewer holes than Carver's. We smell them. They have a funny, musty smell as if they have been in cupboards for a very long time. Valerie, the 'Balcony Boss', wants to know where Sister Morgan has been hiding them all winter. Still we are glad to have an extra blanket.

Carver gets hold of a false rumour. 'I know of some spare hot water bottles,' she whispers to me after supper, very excited. 'Are you sure?' Carver is not always to be trusted in her judgement. 'I promise you I know.' In the lull between day staff going off duty and night staff coming on, we begin to ransack all the cupboards, mostly stuffed with junk, at the bottom of the back stairs. There are no hot water bottles, but we do notice that Valerie seems to be spending an awful lot of time filling up her two. 'She must have got at least six in the bed,' breathes Carver enviously, watching her breath form little clouds in the icy night air. 'She must have found them first.' If only Carver had told me when she first heard about those bottles, we wouldn't be so cold tonight.

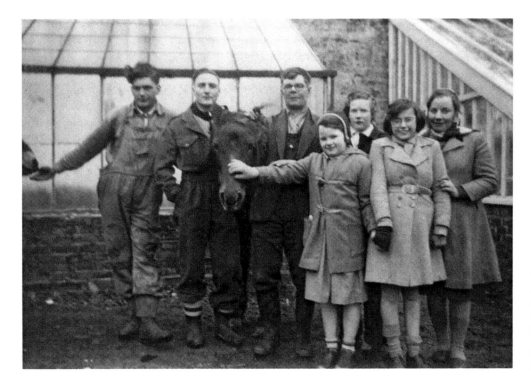

The gardeners, Leslie, Alfie and Arthur feed biscuits to the girls during the cold winter months. The ponies, Lady and Tosca, get in on the act too. Courtesy Christine Perry.

The big freeze

Wednesday, February: Another midweek service. Carver and I make faces at each other behind the vicar's back. It helps to pass the time and take our minds off the extreme cold. He talks about the love of God for his little children, 'Not one sparrow does he see fall but he heeds their suffering. How much more so does he care for you my little children?' We remain unconvinced. Carver and I make ice lollipops on the balcony. The temperature does not rise above freezing all day. Miss White keeps telling us not to worry about the cold because it is good for us. It is all right for her. She does not have to live out on the balcony. We notice that since the temperature dropped below freezing, she no longer bothers to come out through the French doors to see what we are doing. Schoolwork is impossible. Bits of string hold the leaking pieces of tarpaulin to our beds lest they blow off in the icy wind. Each morning we consult the thermometer which hangs over the balcony and inform Miss White of the result. She is not pleased and says she wishes we showed as much interest in our lessons. Finally, I challenge her to read out what it says on the thermometer. 'It's twenty-six degrees Fahrenheit (-3.33º C)!' She refuses to look. Instead, she slaps my face and tells me not to be rude.

Friday morning: I am ill and have been given five big white tablets and told to keep quiet. I think I have a cold in the tummy. Snow covers half my bed and my slippers are soaking from paddling through the wet snow to get inside.

Saturday: I have a temperature of 100 degrees (37.77º C) and I was sick twice in the night. The night nurse never bothered to clean it up and it has frozen. I get up in the afternoon and go with the others for a walk in the snow. We go to the gardeners' shed and sit there for an hour. It's warm and smells earthy. The men are kind and offer us biscuits.

Monday: The temperature falls to twenty degrees F (-6.66º C) and we are given an extra hot water bottle. Where was Sister Morgan hiding them all winter? We don't know. She must have a secret cupboard. Sister Morgan is in a real bad mood because Miss White dared to complain that she too felt cold and why couldn't we have a fire in the ward. It has no heating at all but when the weather gets very, very cold Sister Morgan will allow a small coal fire to be lit. Sister Morgan herself has a one bar electric fire in her office. 'It is impossible to teach when the weather is this cold,' says Miss White. She gets no sympathy from Sister Morgan. 'Go and put on an extra coat instead of moaning to me!' shouts Sister Morgan. 'You are not getting a fire in here, do you hear me? What do you think this place is? If you are not tough enough to stand it then you had better leave!' Miss White goes very quiet. It is silly of Sister Morgan to suggest Miss White put on extra clothing. She is already barely visible under a surfeit of sweaters, woollen stockings, fur lined boots, fur gloves and even a fur hat (we suspect the hat is a gift, or maybe a loan from Dr Hubbard, who seems to own such exotic things). She caps the whole outfit with a very old beaver lamb coat. From her nose hangs a semi-permanent drop. One day, we think it will turn into an icicle. Miss White's pale blue eyes are very watery and she is upset by the extreme temperature and Sister Morgan's lack of sympathy. All this she has to endure in an effort to educate us who do not wish to be educated.

Defeated and humiliated Miss White reappears in the afternoon with a blanket and proceeds to march slowly, funeral like, around the ward. Some girls laugh at this spectacle. Miss White looks like a prisoner. The temperature drops to nineteen degrees F (-7.22º C) and now it is obvious, even to Sister Morgan, that something will have to be done. 'Otherwise we will all perish,' predicts Carver ominously. Carver always looks on the gloomy side of things but on this occasion she might be right. The word goes out that we six on the balcony are going to be moved inside! Great excitement! But first the spare room on Ward 1, the so-called recreation room, though it is never used as such, has to be cleared of junk, and then our six beds are wheeled upstairs. As we help push our beds down the corridor and into the lift, Carver says to me in a whisper, not too loud lest it jeopardize our luck. 'Why couldn't we have been brought in when the temperature first went below zero?' This crosses all our minds though nobody dare raise the question with Sister Morgan. We are too grateful to be inside. The snow continues to fall heavily and we are told that all the roads leading to Craig-y-nos are blocked. And a coal fire is been lit in Ward 2. Miss White sits beside it all day as if her life depends on it. Maybe it does.

The late snowstorm

The first of March brings an unexpected snowstorm and we watch gleefully as the thermometer drops. A month ago we got taken indoors for a week. Only Carver and I are left on the balcony now. The others have been kept indoors for the winter. The snow falls thick and fast, covering the bottom of the beds, then the whole beds and finally the lockers. We put our beds alongside the wall. This gives us some extra protection. Our beds are igloo-like, with bits of old tarpaulin tied with string, which is carefully hoarded for occasions like this. Crawling into bed is a delicate operation. Disrupt the string and there is a bed full of snow. Still, we have had plenty of experience of surviving a night out in the snow so we are not too bothered. Except tonight, there is an unexpected turn of events.

There is a new night nurse called Molly Evans. She's young and innocent of the ways of Craig-y-nos and this is her first winter here. 'You poor things,' she murmurs when she comes on duty and peers at us through the French doors. 'I can't leave you out here all night.' Actually, we are quite comfortable by now and have warmed up with our extra hot water bottles, collected from Sarah who went home last week, and extra blankets from Mavis who seems to have disappeared to another hospital. 'I will pull your beds into the ward for the night,' she says. We are surprised and delighted, though we dare not tell her that Sister Morgan will be in a really bad temper when she comes on duty the following morning. Carver and I make the most of the occasion. We entertain Ward 2 by dancing on the table and having races, leaping from bed to bed around the ward. Carver wins, to my annoyance. It is a lively and very noisy night and we have great fun. It is short lived. The night orderly, who hears all the rumpus, reports us to day staff, and the new young nurse Molly Evans is exceedingly hurt and angry when she comes on duty the following night. By this time we have been pushed back onto the balcony, very unceremoniously, by Sister Morgan. 'A bit of snow has never harmed anyone,' she says, shoving our beds into the white fluffy stuff which has now settled into a thick carpet over the cemented balcony floor. 'You are not grateful for the favours I do you,' says Nurse Evans, and scolds us. She's hurt. We feel sorry she got into trouble.

The hygiene lesson

Miss White slaps my face during the hygiene lesson. 'You are making fun of the subject! It is very important.' It's true. We mock hygiene lessons, which are all about diagrams of germs walking around. Each week we get a hygiene lesson, along with a religious service. We are told all about germs and how to get rid of them so that when we leave and grow up we will know how to be clean, then we won't be ill again. Well, Miss White gets to the section on 'How germs enter the body,' and she explains at great length to the whole of the ward. She stands in the doorway between the balcony and Ward 2 so that everyone has the benefit of her knowledge. 'On no account, girls, are you to stick pins into your hands. This will allow the germs to get in. Turn to page eleven in your hygiene book, girls!' We do as we were told. 'Now, you can see from these illustrations how the germs walk in through the pin holes.' 'How many legs have the germs got?' I ask. Miss White goes very red in the face and comes over and slaps me. She is quite angry.

Carver giggles. 'Look, the germs in my book have got more legs than Ann's. Will they walk faster?' Carver gets slapped in the face too. Miss White tells us not to drink milk with flies in it, 'Even if you take the flies out first. Remember, girls, it does not matter if you pull the flies out or not. The germs remain,' says Miss White in her high squeaky voice. We do not care for hygiene lessons.

Night beauty

Night sister Thomas catches two girls kissing behind a locker in Ward 2, and scolds them. 'It's very unhygienic! Don't ever let me catch you doing it again! Very unhygienic, do you understand?' We hear the commotion from the balcony and we rush to stuff all our books, curlers and torches under the bedclothes ready for her nightly inspection. She comes out on to the balcony, somewhat distraught by her discovery, and stands staring at the mountains, hardly casting a glance in our direction. The staff take a dim view of girls behaving badly. We pretend to be asleep though she knows perfectly well we are only pretending. It is a glorious night with a full moon and the place looks particularly beautiful, not that we much bothered about such things, having more immediate concerns to worry about. 'The trouble with you lot," says Sister Thomas, turning sharply to face us, 'is that you are incapable of appreciating beauty.' With that she stalks off indoors.

'Stupid woman,' says Carver, 'always staring at the mountains!' 'What does she expect us to do? Sing to them?' says I, who hates singing. 'She's horrible. She shouts at us even when we haven't done anything wrong,' says Elspeth, the quiet one, and the newest on the balcony. Suddenly, there is an uneasy murmur from the bed nearest the French doors and a shadow moves away. It is Sister Thomas.

Trapped in lift

An uneasy relationship exists between Sister Winnie Morgan and Dr Hubbard. They share little in common, except that both work at Craig-y-nos and both are women, though 'woman' is not a word often used to describe Dr Hubbard. Indeed, one child insists she's a man. Her gender does cause confusion in the minds of small children.

One day, Dr Hubbard gets stuck in the lift, a huge ancient contraption more like a cage than a device for moving people, dead and alive, between floors. The gates refuse to open. She rattles them, and the noise brings Sister Morgan from her office who seeing her plight, bursts out laughing. 'Get me out of here!' shouts Dr Hubbard. Sister Morgan screeches. All this noise brings us racing out of Ward 2 down the corridor to see what all the fuss is about. 'A shilling to view, girls!' says Sister Morgan and titters at her own joke. Dr Hubbard begins shouting in a foreign language. We are transfixed. We have never heard another tongue spoken before. 'I knew you reminded me of something,' says Sister Morgan. 'I can see it now. You must be very closely related to a monkey, much closer than the rest of us.' It's true. Dr Hubbard looks like a caged monkey, but unlike a monkey, she is not going to remain in the lift forever.

Sister Morgan forgets this. She is too busy enjoying the moment. Dr Hubbard becomes extremely vociferous, shouting even louder. Whatever she is saying about Sister Morgan, we fear it is not complimentary. Nurse Glenys Davies appears. She suggests that Sister Morgan ring for the hospital engineer. She does, reluctantly, and emerges a few minutes later from her office, triumphant. 'He's in Cardiff for the day. You know the rules.' Nobody except the hospital engineer is allowed to touch the lift. So what to do? Sister Morgan is all for leaving Dr Hubbard there for the rest of the day, but Nurse Davies intervenes. She offers to try and free Dr Hubbard. First, we are shooed back to our ward because it is not appropriate for us to be relishing Dr Hubbard's embarrassment and imprisonment. Nevertheless, we continue to peep through the glass door of Ward 2 as Dr Hubbard paces up and down inside the lift. Indeed, like a caged gorilla. It takes a long time, despite Nurse Glenys Davies' efforts, before she is freed. Sister Morgan, we note, does not help. Rather, she stands there offering advice. For the rest of the day though, Sister Morgan is in very high spirits, and to celebrate, she puts Thomas, the hospital cat, in our food cupboard.

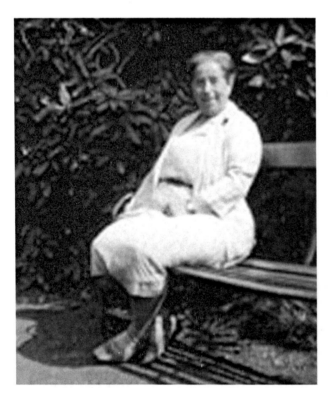

Dr Hubbard's approach to the children was described by school inspectors in 1946 as 'Not always too gentle in manner'. Courtesy Ann Shaw.

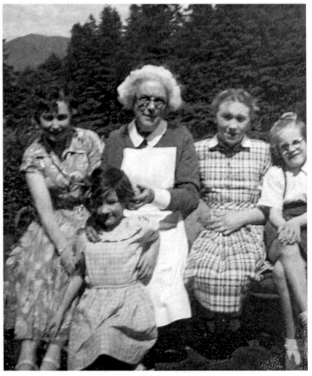

Sister Morgan with young patients. Between her and Dr Hubbard there was a 'battle of wills'. Courtesy Molly Barry.

A special treat for Thomas

Our food cupboard is in the side kitchen next to the bathroom, and it's here that staff make tea and snacks for us. It contains our weekly rations, mostly fish paste, bread, butter, biscuits, one big lump of cheese and a fruitcake. The mice are very fond of this cupboard, too, and sometimes we find their tiny teeth marks in our cheese, or hear them scampering around. Sister Morgan rattles the bathroom door. 'Come and see Thomas mousing, girls!'

Washing is a communal event, an evening ritual as we queue to use the single washbasin. Missing your place can mean another ten minutes or longer to wait. Still, an order from Sister Morgan must be obeyed. We troop out in our dressing gowns, clutching our flannels, soap and towels. 'Who's going to catch all those mice that have been nibbling away at our rations?' murmurs Sister Morgan, stroking the delighted Thomas as he purrs his way around the cupboard, stacked with plates of bread and butter, buns and jam. We watch in silence. We pretend to be impressed with Thomas' antics though secretly we are a bit shocked and wish he would finish so we can go back to our washing. Thomas is not to be hurried. Such treats do not come his way every day. He sniffs at the plates, raises his nose delicately, and walks between them until he comes to our weekly cake. But, he decides it's too stale for him, for after a quick lick he continues his perambulations between the dishes. He shows not the least bit of interest in the pot of jam or the fish-paste - another weekly treat - nor a large chunk of cheese, which the mice have already tucked into. But he does stop at a big mouse-hole.

'Watch him, girls. This is it! Thomas is the best mouser we've ever had,' says Sister Morgan. We say nothing. Any mouse with an ounce of sense would never leave the security of its nest to step into a cupboard with a big fat black cat waiting on the other side. Thomas thinks so too. He gets up, bored, and he is about to leap out of the cupboard when he sees something he does like. Our milk jug. He drops his tongue into it. 'Oooh, naughty pussy! Haven't I told you before that you must not drink milk out of the jug?' We watch in silence. 'Ooh, naughty pussy!' she repeats, but does not stop him. 'Isn't he a greedy cat, girls?' She turns to us for approval. We nod. Thomas gets extra rations from somewhere. Cats don't grow to that size on hospital food. 'I have fed him twice today and he's still hungry.' 'More like three times,' whispers Carver. We note that Sister Morgan leaves Thomas lapping the milk for a long time before picking him up. Still, it's good to see her in such a good mood so we accept Thomas 'mousing' in our food cupboard and go back to our washing.

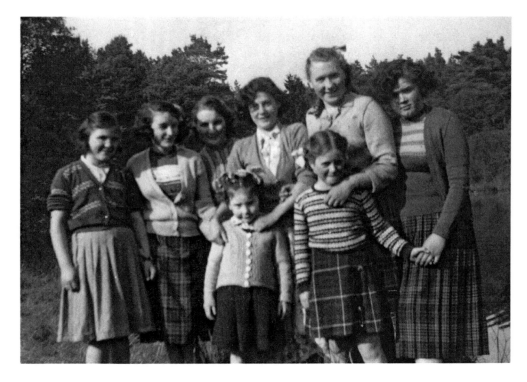

'Up' children (those not on bed rest) were allowed to walk in the grounds during the afternoons. By the early 1950s, boys who were 'up' were moved to Highland Moors, Llandrindod Wells. Courtesy Ann Shaw.

The singing lesson

Every afternoon between two and four o'clock we are allowed to go for a walk in the castle grounds. We have a secret venue, one that the staff never suspect so they can't forbid us to go there. We walk straight to the gardeners' shed where we sit on wooden orange boxes and watch the men while they brew tea and eat their sandwiches. Sometimes, they share a piece of cake with us or give us a biscuit. The older girls like to flirt with the men while the young ones, like Carver and myself, just sit and watch. Sometimes, we stay in the shed, which is warm and smells very earthy, for over an hour while all the time Dr Hubbard, Sister Morgan and Miss White think we are filling our lungs with fresh air.

One Thursday afternoon we are on our way back from the gardeners' shed ready for the weekly three o'clock singing lesson when Valerie, the new 'Balcony Boss', says, 'Let's not go back to singing! Let's go and hide in the shrubbery.' 'Yippee!' yell Carver and myself. We hate singing. All six of us scramble amongst the rhododendrons. It's dark and mysterious in here. We pick snow drops because it's spring, and we giggle and chew leaves and wonder if they are poisonous, and if so will we die. At three o clock Miss White appears on the balcony of Ward 2. We watch from the security of the dense shrubbery. 'Girls, girls! Where are you? It's time for your singing lesson.' She calls in vain. I part the leaves to get a better view, only to find myself smacked by Valerie. 'Do you want her to see us?' she hisses. Carver starts giggling and Rosie announces she is peeing herself with excitement. It's all a test of Valerie's authority. 'Get behind those rocks if you can't control yourself! And you, Rosie, go and pee somewhere out of sight.' If Miss White had been wearing her correct spectacles, which she isn't because she is always losing them, she couldn't but fail to see us for all the commotion we are making.

Later we overhear Miss White grumbling to Sister Morgan. 'The girls won't come back for their singing lessons.' Sister Morgan shows not the least sympathy. 'Don't blame them,' she laughs and walks away. But Miss White reports us to Dr Hubbard and that's the last time we are allowed out on a Thursday.

Miss White's breakdown

It is a Wednesday morning and we are waiting for the doctors to do their Long Round, so called because they take such a long time to go around each bed. We hate Long Round because we have to sit by our beds, if we are up, and those in bed have to remain immobile, like little corpses, making certain that all signs of their daily life are removed. Everything must be spotless, tidy, with no sign of human activity. We remain like this for maybe two hours. Dr Williams accompanied by Dr Hubbard and Sister Morgan go to each bed, talk about the person in it as if they are invisible, then move on. It's all very boring. Sometimes, after these visits we are sent for X-rays, visits to the dentist, or worse, ordered to have another lot of injections and PAS, a horrible tasting medicine.

Well, we are all sitting by our beds out on the balcony when the word is flashed to us that Miss White has walked out, tears running down her face. 'I can't stand it any longer! You are all driving me mad. I am going to leave before it is too late.' But of course it's too late. Far too late for her, Dr Hubbard, Sister Morgan, and other single members of staff to leave Craig-y-nos. This is their life. They are held in invisible chains within the castle, any dream of a normal life gone long ago. For us though there is hope that one day we will be free. The news of Miss White's breakdown causes a ripple of alarm to spread through Ward 2. Carver and I run inside to find out the source of the commotion. 'What's happened? What is it?' 'It's her,' says Vera, the 'Ward Boss', pointing at Rachel, a malevolent fifteen-year-old, unpopular with everyone. 'She made fun of Miss White being a spinster,' cried Rosie. 'You shouldn't have said it,' shouted Vera. 'It's true,' says Rachel, unrepentant and glad of the stir she had caused, for now she is the centre of attention.

But Vera smells trouble. 'Where's Miss White?' 'Sitting in the chair next to the lift,' says Carver. 'Just what I thought!' says Vera. 'She has pulled this trick before. She's waiting for the doctors. Any minute now the lift gates will open with them all inside.' She turns to Carver and myself. 'Go and apologize to Miss White!' We object vociferously. 'But we didn't make her cry! We were not even in the room at the time.' 'That's not the point. Get down there and talk to her! If Dr Hubbard finds Miss White crying, we are going to get into the most awful trouble.' We had only popped into the ward to see what was going on and now we are being ordered to apologize for something we didn't do or even see happen. But Vera is right. We walk down the corridor and Miss White is so surprised to see us that she dabs her eyes and stops crying. 'The ward wants you to know that they are sorry and will you please return,' we say. She needs little persuasion. Like us, she knows the outcome will be very serious if Dr Hubbard discovers that we made her cry. Miss White re-enters Ward 2 and Vera gives a fulsome apology on behalf of the ward. Rachel, much to her chagrin, is ordered to say sorry. She only just finishes when the lift gates clank open.

The forbidden film

Dr Hubbard got it into her head we are hoarding handkerchiefs in our lockers, so she orders a search to be carried out. Our lockers are emptied and all handkerchiefs burnt. They find six. Dr Hubbard then issues a brisk order, 'Nobody under eighteen-years-of-age can go the pictures next Monday. The film is unsuitable for children.' That's us. Ward 2. Well, those seven of us who are up and about. The rest, who are in bed, don't count. Carver and I are intrigued. What could it possibly be? 'Let's go and find out,' says Carver on the Monday afternoon. We sneak down the stairs and creep up to the door of the Patti theatre. Carver puts her ear against it. She is very good at door-listening, though not much use these days for breaking into the library since she put on two pounds. 'Is it sex?' says I, thinking this will be a subject of which Dr Hubbard would most certainly not approve. Carver shakes her head. 'Seems like some kind of a fight. I can't tell.' 'We are going to have to open the door,' says Carver. 'Watch it! It squeaks.'

As Carver edges open the door, it makes a heavy groan followed by a deep squeak. Luckily, this is lost in the shriek coming from the cinema screen. 'Murder!' breathe Carver and I together. It's the first time we have seen one human being kill another, even if it is only on screen. We watch as a man plunges a knife into the prostrate body of a woman half-lying in her bed and half falling out. The knife goes deep into the woman's back. Her shrieks as she lies dying cause us to step back sharply and close the door, but not before we catch sight of Dr Hubbard sitting in her usual leather chair, her thick lips parted with excitement and her eyes transfixed on the screen. 'So that's what she didn't want us to see,' whispers Carver. I nod. We might have guessed. We are not surprised that Dr Hubbard enjoys violence.

The missing parcel

Mabel, the cleaner, tells me there is a parcel for me in the office. I want it but Sister Morgan is holding on to it. 'How can I let Sister Morgan know that I have found out?' I ask Carver. 'Tell her you are expecting a parcel from your mother because she promised you a new jumper, and you are cold and waiting for it to arrive.' I am not so sure. My clothes have been the subject of some dispute between Dr Hubbard and my mother. A few months ago I was told to write home and tell mother to bring me in some clothes because I was going to be allowed up. So a parcel arrived, and for the first time in two years I had proper clothes to wear. I remember the excitement when Sister Morgan handed me the parcel, already opened, as it was the custom to search everything. And the feeling of slight disappointment that mother had sent me grey clothes - a grey skirt, grey twinset and grey socks. I had hoped, indeed expected, a bit of colour. However, I was delighted to have proper clothes again and put them on feeling very proud. No doubt I looked a bit peculiar, like an orphan in institutional clothing. Not that it bothered me, though I could see that I was dressed differently from the other girls. However, it bothered Dr Hubbard, for on the next visiting my mother was ordered to go and see her. A rare event. 'She says I must get you some clothes suitable for a little girl, not grey. You must have clothes with colour in them.' Shortly after that, a red sweater arrived.

After the fracas over my clothes, I think it unlikely that Sister Morgan will believe mother has sent me another jumper. One is enough. Sometimes though she sends me sweets, or even as a special treat, a box of chocolates. This is what Mabel has reported seeing in Sister Morgan's office. Now, we have long had our suspicions that Sister Morgan keeps our parcels for days before handing them over. She will say that she had to search them for improper food, though why this search should sometimes take a week, is beyond us. Once, Vera, the 'Ward Boss' challenges her, demanding to know outright if her mother has sent a parcel for her birthday. She had, and the result was that Sister Morgan held onto it for another day. So I decide that it will be better to keep quiet and wait with growing excitement for the parcel, knowing it is there, in Sister Morgan's office. Two days later Sister Morgan hands me my parcel. It is, indeed, a box of chocolates, a magazine on budgies, and a new vest. Everything had been opened, including the box of chocolates (only three missing) and the letter from mother.

Each morning we consult
the thermometer which hangs
over the balcony and inform
Miss White of the result.

She is not pleased and says
she wishes we showed as much
interest in our lessons. Finally,
I challenge her to read out what
it says on the thermometer. 'It's
twenty-six degrees Fahrenheit
(-3.33^{o} C)!' She refuses to look.

Instead, she slaps my face
and tells me not to be rude.

Ann Shaw (Rumsey)

Tadpoles

The snow's gone and more girls have been pushed out on to the balcony for the 'spring air'. I've collected water for my tadpoles from the lake in the grounds. Mavis, the orderly, tells me that the way to keep my tadpoles alive is to give them water from the lake. I had used tap water and they had all died. Mavis knows about such things from her children. So, I go over with three jars and fill them up. Unfortunately, I fill them up too much, and I spill some of it as I pass Miss White who is standing in her usual position just inside the French doors, trying to instill some kind of education into us while at the same time (more pertinent to her), keeping herself warm. It is not a pretty sight. Anyway, I spill some of my precious lake water as I pass her because I am nervous and know that she does not approve of my tadpoles or slugs, which I gather and keep on my locker in big bell jars brought in by Mavis. Something her children have once used. Miss White hits me on the head which causes me to spill even more water. 'Tell me, when are you going home?' I don't care for the tone of her voice. It is as if she is anxious to see the back of me, which I dare say she is.

Two years on - the relapse

Now I have a name for him, the man I had known only as the 'X-ray man' thanks to the recollections of Joan Collins (Coughlan). He's called Mr Hughes and he came from Swansea to do the X-rays at Craig-y-nos. My memory of him is not pleasant though I hasten to add through no fault of his. More a case of circumstances, and the way it was in those days. Mr Hughes probably never even gave it a thought, except perhaps to comment later in the day, maybe to his wife, that there had been an incident with a difficult child.

My best friend Rosemary has just gone home and I am told by Sister Morgan that if my X-ray is okay then I, too, will be going home. After more than two years in Craig-y-nos I skip down to the X-ray department. X-rays are a routine feature of life every three months (if I remember correctly). This is long before the dangers of radiation became known. Automatically, I go through the standard procedure. 'Take your clothes off ... stand there ... take a deep breath.' Click. Off to get dressed. Only this time, as I am in the middle of dressing, I am told to wait. A nurse appears with a worried look on her face. The 'X-ray man' stands in the doorway. 'There's a problem. We need to do more X-rays. We need to do a tomograph. We need deeper X-rays.' They don't need to spell it out. I know the scene. I've got TB again. I've had a relapse. Back to bed with PAS and injections. No going home.

I cry, I howl in protest. A nurse sits me down in the waiting room. She puts her arm around me. I refuse to be comforted. The more she hugs and talks to me the worse I get. The X-ray man says he can't do the X-rays with the state I am in. They go into a huddle. It's nearly midday. They walk me into the X-ray room and I am told to climb up and lie down on the X-ray machine. It is a tomogram. A blanket is thrown over me. Nothing is said, or if it is I am too distressed to hear it. They walk out and close the door. They go for dinner. I am alone for an hour, maybe longer. I have no memory of time except that I know I am alone in this room full of machines, and it's hard lying on this slab of metal. My sobbing eventually wears itself out and by the time they return it's given way to sniveling, broken by the occasional gut-wrenching sob (to this day the sound of children crying sends a cold chill through me). The tomograph over, I am wheeled back to Ward 2, humiliated.

Many years later I revisit Craig-y-nos. I am shown the derelict X-ray department and I stare at the empty space which once housed the X-ray machines. My guide, a young girl from the Rhondda Valley, interrupts my reverie. She points to a bricked up door, 'That led straight to the morgue.' The grotesque horror of the situation finally hits me. During that hour that I had been left alone in the X-ray department, weeping, I was in fact not alone. I had some silent companions only yards away. Very silent.

Three years on - the Box Room

I am still on the balcony, except some winters I am taken indoors if it gets very cold. I caught TB again about a year ago, just as I was ready to go home. So, here I am back on injections and medicine again. I prefer the balcony. We have more freedom. We are seven girls on the balcony. Rita, who has been living in the corner for over a year, got into the habit of playing with herself during the day and Nurse Evans keeps catching her at it. 'I will tie your hands to the side of the bed if I see you at it again!' she shouts at poor Rita. Sometimes, Auntie Maggie takes pity on her and gives her a sweet if she happens to have some in her pocket.

Rita's family visit on rare occasions. Nurse Evans' threats have no effect on her because she is a bit simple, and playing with herself is her only pleasure, so they move her indoors in order to keep an eye on her. The staff hope to cure her of the habit by shouting at her. It doesn't work so they move her to the Box Room, so called because it looks like a square box.

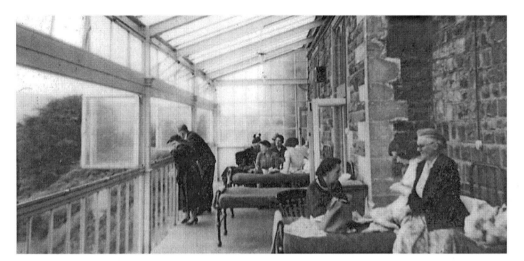

Balcony life may have been cold but the children enjoyed the 'freedom'. Being confined to the 'Box Room' was considered a dreadful punishment. Courtesy Christine Perry.

Suzie's night of passion

The older girls talk a lot about sex, men and marriage. They want to know what goes on in the bedroom - well, the bed to be exact. One of the married orderlies, Suzie, will often oblige. Sometimes, Jean and Valerie, both aged fifteen, will give Suzie sweets or even a piece of chocolate to encourage her to go into more details.

One morning, throughout breakfast, Suzie keeps hinting that something special had happened to her the night before. While serving out the morning porridge, grey, lumpy, lukewarm and sprinkled with stuff that looks like ground up cardboard to encourage us to eat more, she keeps rolling her eyes around and whispering to Valerie that she has something to tell her. Even I am curious. 'Come on then, Suzie, tell us all about it,' urges Valerie. A ripple of giggling breaks out amongst the eight dressing-gowned clad girls, the only ones allowed up. Space is made on the bed for Suzie to sit, and the rest of us scramble for a position as best we can. Suzie raises her hand. This is the signal for us all to stop talking. She wants absolute silence before she begins her story. It always starts the same. How her husband strokes her back, then her throat, followed by her breasts and … Valerie interrupts. 'Look, we've heard all this before.' But Suzie ignores Valerie and carries on with her story. It is always the same. Suzie likes sex yet she appears to like the preliminaries even more.

This is in marked contrast to Edith, another orderly. She dislikes sex and says it is something 'Women have got to put up with if they want a husband.' Now, this doesn't seem to fit with Suzie's experience, where she can't get enough of it. Edith often tells us about her honeymoon night, 'He woke me in the middle of the night to do it and I was tired after a day's travelling.' Sex never pleases Edith so we listen quietly while Suzie goes into all the details. When Valerie thinks that Suzie has indulged herself enough, she tries to hurry the story on. 'Let's hear the interesting bit now Suzie. Y'know, when he climbs …' She offers Suzie an apple. Suzie takes it, sniffs it twice then wipes it on her apron. It looks like a sweet apple and I am surprised to see Valerie parting with it so easily. Suzie too appreciates this unexpected gift and begins eating it. 'What was it like?' demands Valerie. 'Ooh, it was lovely,' murmurs Suzie, hugging herself and eating her apple at the same time. She seems lost in a world of rapture, of which we know nothing. 'What was lovely?' demands Janet, the practical one. 'You know what I mean,' says Suzie, rolling her eyes. 'That's it, we don't,' says Jean. 'We want you to tell us.'

'He stuck it in so hard that I didn't know where I was.' This is not particularly helpful. In fact, it is most disappointing. Valerie says afterwards that she regrets giving Suzie the apple. She only has three left and visiting is not for another two weeks.

Sexual experiments in Ward 2

All this talk of sex arouses Valerie and Jean's curiosity even more. That night they decide to find out for themselves. After lights out they put the screens around Valerie's bed and Jean climbs in. We all know what is going on and shout words of encouragement. 'How are you supposed to lie?' asks eleven-year-old Elsie, peeping through the curtains. 'Get out!' shrieks Valerie. 'This is private! You must not watch.' 'Get back to your bed,' orders Josephine, the 'Ward Boss'. 'If I catch you peeping again, I will get out of bed and thrash you myself.' She's been on total bed rest for more than a year but is not averse to leaping out of bed and marching around if she thinks her authority is being undermined. Elsie creeps back to bed. 'Your turn will come one day,' promises Josephine. 'What for?' asks Elsie. Josephine ignores the question. Everyone is too busy listening to what is going on behind the screen.

Valerie and Jean quarrel. They both wanted to be the man. Valerie, who is stronger and more aggressive, and a year older, wins that battle. Jean does not take kindly to being told to lie on her back and open her legs. They suspect they are missing something but they aren't sure what. It is this 'something' that seems to produce waves of ecstasy in Suzie. 'How about a banana?' shouts Josephine. The consensus from the ward is that a banana will be suitable. Who has one left? Usually, they get eaten within days of visiting. 'I think Rachel has still got some bananas in her locker?' says Josephine. Rachel says nothing. She does indeed have bananas and she is reluctant to part with them. It is another two weeks to visiting. 'How many have you got?' demands Josephine. 'Two,' says Rachel timidly. 'You don't need two bananas! Go on throw one over.' Rachel does as she is told. It goes over the screen and lands on the floor. Valerie has to get out of bed and that gets her into a bad mood. 'I was just getting into the swing of it,' she shouts. When Jean sees the size of the banana she squeals. 'You're not putting that up me!' She objects to the size. So Rachel gets her banana back. Instead, the pair of them resort to jigging up and down in the bed and we can hear the bed springs going so fast that we think they will break. They try very hard to reach this world of ecstasy that Suzie speaks so lovingly about, but they fail. Next day, they tell Suzie about their love-making but she is unable to tell them where they had gone wrong.

Last year in Craig-y-nos - Bullying on the balcony

'It's your turn to be 'Balcony Boss',' the girls chant. 'I don't want to be.' 'You've got to. You're the oldest.' Custom is that the oldest girl in the ward or balcony becomes the 'Boss'. Suddenly it's my turn. Gwen, age fifteen, has gone home. Now, at thirteen-years-of-age, I am the next oldest, but I don't want the job. I don't want to boss around the younger children for I am still a child myself. I am thirteen and four months but I am still nine, the age I was when I came into Craig-y-nos. I haven't moved on. I have lived for almost four years on one floor of the castle, going out at set times for a few hours in the grounds, but only since I have been allowed up. So, the next girl in age, Mary, gets the job.

Then it starts. Someone snatches a book I am reading. *Girl*, my favourite comic, along with *Children's Weekly Newspaper*, disappears. What's happening? I don't understand. I ask questions. They ignore me. And the dentist gives me a brace to wear because I have big gaps where he has taken teeth out. He decides the answer is to fill the gaps by pulling the teeth together because I look like a mini vampire. I am ugly and getting uglier by the day as my body is changing and I don't know what to do about it. I have to take my dental brace out to eat. So, I leave it in the cubbyhole of my locker. It's an extraordinary pink and metal contraption. Except one day, I go back on to the balcony and it's gone. Panic! Search. Nowhere to be found. I report the loss to Sister Morgan. She tells Dr Hubbard who punishes me. 'No more walks, or going to the cinema until you find it.' And the girls aren't talking to me now. Isolated.

Monday afternoon they go to the film show. I stay alone on my bed on the balcony. That's when I make the next discovery. My precious box of ribbons, the only thing I possess in Craig-y-nos that I am most proud of, has disappeared. My world disintegrates. I can take no more. I run to the only place I know that I will be secure. The turret room in the castle, a secret place I go to read, and I cry and cry, for hours. The only time I have cried since I was told, two years ago, that I had a relapse and had to go back to bed. Four o'clock, the girls return. I hear them shouting my name. Eventually, they find me. Auntie Maggie is with them. She puts her arm around me. This sets me off crying even more. I find myself apologizing, though wonder what on earth for? I have done no wrong. Yet, it is my way of ingratiating myself back into the group. I want to be liked by them. I want them to be my friends. So I have to grovel and say I am sorry. And my box of ribbons re-appears along with other books, and even my favourite pencil. But no dental brace. A few weeks later I go home, and a couple of months afterwards the postman delivers a strange little package to the farm. It's from Sister Morgan and contains my dental brace. She says the girls found it in the rhododendron bushes.

Great news

Hurray! It's definite! I am told that I am to go home. After all this time, nearly four years, I can't believe it. But it's true. I am beside myself with excitement. It seems that my last X-rays were satisfactory and I am to go home in a few weeks time. What will home be like? Mother has been sent for and told the news. Dr Williams, the head doctor, is going to inspect the farmhouse to see that it is suitable for me to live in. Mother reports after the next visiting that Dr Williams has visited and he does not like the stream running through the middle of the 'big kitchen', though mother explains that it only happens when it rains very hard, and she always takes up the rugs. Unfortunately, it is raining when Dr Williams visits and she has the rugs all piled up in a corner. He gets his feet wet stepping across the stream to the parlour, which mother says I can use as a bedroom. Dr Williams tells them they must do something about the state of the farmhouse. That it is too damp for me to return to. She tells him that people have lived like this in Ty-Llangenny for nearly five hundred years and what was alright for my ancestors surely will be alright for me now that I am well again. They are told to cement the floor so that the stream will be hidden and this is going to take a few weeks. Mother says it's such a fuss having me coming home and she has such a lot to do with early spring lambing. She hints to the doctors that I might stay in until the summer.

Will I recognize my brother, David, eighteen months younger than me? I saw him once, six months after I had been in, when a nurse lifted me to the window to see him in the courtyard. It was difficult to make him out amongst all the people there. He waved. It's such a long time that I have only vague memories of what it is to live in a family. Mother says she is going to buy me a Corgi puppy. I don't know what a Corgi looks like so I break into the library and find a book on dogs. A Corgi is a dog with short legs, long body and no tail. Snaps at cows heels.

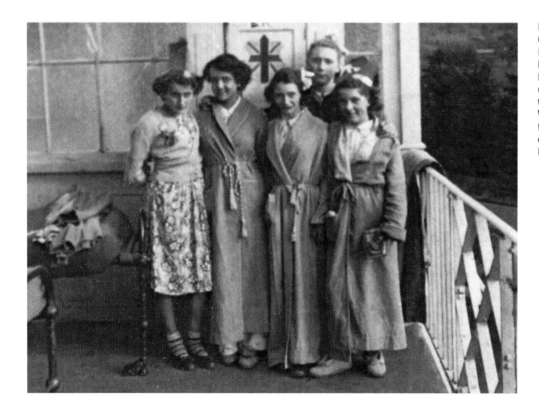

Left to right: Barbara O'Connell (Paines), Florence, Ann Shaw (Rumsey), Mari Friend (Jenkins) and unidentified celebrate the Coronation, 1953. Ward 2 balcony is festooned with decorations. Courtesy Mari Friend.

Going home

Mother says the 'big kitchen' has a new floor made from cement, and she has put rugs on it bought from Abergavenny market with the money she has saved from selling her eggs. She says it looks 'very smart'. They have even installed an indoor lavatory with a proper chain and water. The parlour has been converted into a bedroom for me and I will have a fire in it too! Mother says she has bought me some new furniture - my own wardrobe, dressing-table and a locker.

After four years it all seems like a dream. I can't believe it. I can't sleep at night for the excitement and I have started to give away 'keepsakes', a ritual for all girls leaving - a slide here, a comb there, a ribbon. Finally, the dawn breaks for the last time for me in Craig-y-nos Castle. I am wide awake and watch the sun rise, so nervous with excitement at the thought of going home again. Mother has promised me a puppy, a little Corgi dog that will be all mine and is waiting for me. He is called Bonnie. In the morning, I thank Dr Hubbard, Sister Morgan and Miss White for all they have done for me. This is a custom. Then, just before mother arrives - as soon as the word has flashed around that the car has driven in through the gates to collect me - I rush around each bed giving every girl a quick, legitimate kiss. Half an hour later (why did it take so much time for mother and the relatives to bid farewell to Sister Morgan?), I leave amidst tears and frantic waving of hands, and promises to write. The iron gates of Craig-y-nos slam behind me after four years and three days.

Everyone in the car - crammed with relations whom I have never seen before - is strangely silent as mother drives through the Brecon Beacons back to Ty-Llangenny Farm, near Crickhowell, a home which is just a vague memory. The delay in my departure and the silence in the car, I later learn, is because the relations were busy demanding of Dr Hubbard and Sister Morgan that I be kept in Craig-y-nos a bit longer.

Epilogue

I had so looked forward to going home but nothing prepares me for the disappointment and sense of alienation that follows, for I had left Ty-Llangenny Farm a child and returned a teenager. Suddenly, the outside world is a frightening place. I miss Craig-y-nos and cry each night wanting to go back, yet know I can't. Those first few weeks at home are painful. I hate it! I hate being singled out as 'the sick child'. People come to visit and stare at me as if I was some strange creature - lowered voices and whispering when they look at me. One aunt says in a loud voice, 'You would have thought they would have kept her there until she was cured.' Mother intervenes, 'She has just got a bit of a cold.' My aunt is unconvinced. She keeps away from me. She refuses to eat at our table, even to drink a cup of tea lest she 'catch something,' I hear her whisper to my father. All I want is the company of the girls and the security of Craig-y-nos. At least I knew who I was and my place in that cloistered world. Here on the farm I find myself relegated to an invalid. Yet how could this be? Had I not been one of the fittest at Craig-y-nos.

Worse is to come when I start school, a local convent, because I am judged too delicate to go to the secondary modern. But it gives me a private education, an opportunity to catch up on my lost schooling that will one day lead to a fistful of certificates and my passport out of Wales. The girls in the convent in Abergavenny mock my accent. They talk 'posh' and some parents even pay for their daughters to talk 'posher' by sending them for elocution lessons. My years in Craig-y-nos have given me a strong Welsh valleys accent. Again, there is the problem of not knowing what standard of education I have reached. During the interview, the head teacher, a nun with a stern eye, asks me to do some mental arithmetic, some tables. I have never learnt tables in my life. Miss White thought them pointless. 'What are seven eights?' The head nun fixes her watery blue eyes on me. She might just as well have asked me to explain the laws of physics. So, I am put in the B stream, the stream for duffers. At the end of the first term, a ripple of shock goes round the class when class positions are announced. I am first. I don't know who is most surprised, the teachers, pupils or myself. So, I get moved up a class.

Finally, the outside world begins to make sense. There is hope. I am not stupid. It is just that I have never had any formal education. Moreover, I enjoy learning. Going into shops is another revelation. I make the mistake of going into the local ironmongers and asking for toothpaste, and the strange looks I get from the assistant. Mother explains that different shops sell different things, not like our shop at Craig-y-nos (the one from which Carver and I, as errand girls, got sacked), which sold everything - well everything that was deemed suitable. I have to learn to live in a family again, to get to know my brother, to sit at a table and eat properly. For I have become institutionalized, if not semi-feral. After I have been home for a month, mother takes me back to visit Craig-y-nos. She thinks this will cure me of my homesickness for the castle. This is a bad experience, and I had so looked forward to seeing my friends again. I have changed. They haven't. They are still lying in their beds, and I am out in a very different world, a world I can no longer share with them, neither do I yet feel part of. I am in limbo.

Ann became a newspaper journalist. She is married, lives in Scotland and works as a freelance writer/artist.

Teenagers' Stories

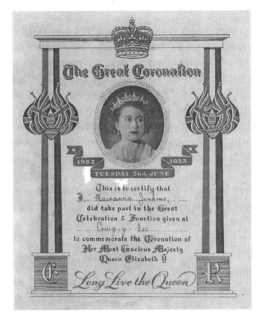

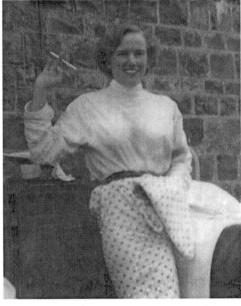

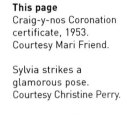

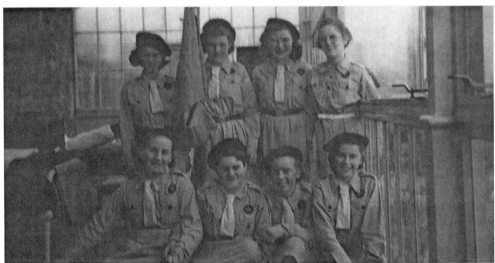

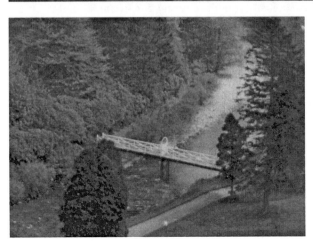

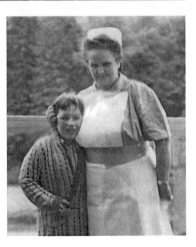

This page
Craig-y-nos Coronation certificate, 1953. Courtesy Mari Friend.

Sylvia strikes a glamorous pose. Courtesy Christine Perry.

Craig-y-nos Girl Guides. The group was established and captained by Ina Hopkins, one of the hospital secretaries and an ex-patient. Christine is holding the standard (back row, left). Courtesy Christine Perry.

Bridge over the River Tawe seen from the Castle balconies. Courtesy Mari Friend.

Auntie Maggie with a boy from Ward 1. From Auntie Maggie's personal collection.

Opposite page
Marlene in the 'Six-bedder' (Adelina Patti's boudoir) with a visiting relative. Courtesy Marlene Philibosian.

Auntie Maggie with Molly Barry. Auntie Maggie was a friend to children and adults alike. From Auntie Maggie's personal collection.

Marlene Philibosian (Hopkins) – The frozen twin-set

I live in California and every now and again I type 'Craig-y-nos' into Google, perhaps out of nostalgia. Well, I got quite a shock when I saw a picture of my bed on the web! I was on Ward 2, on blocks, right by the window. I was there from 1953 for two years from about fourteen or fifteen years of age. I had streptomycin. The isolation from the family was the biggest adjustment, and I still have the letter they wrote to my mother saying I was ready to be picked up.

I remember lying in bed and looking out of the window across to the farm. There was a cow in the field and I thought that cow was mine. I collected stamps. I read a lot. It has made me appreciate that I can be by myself and still enjoy that. It made me independent. I read the Bible daily and I do believe it sustained me and gave me hope. I still have a diary from Craig-y-nos. I took my temperature and pulse and I would record that and other silly little things, including Sister Morgan's mood. I put in my diary the only time she smiled was the day she told me I was going home. Thank God for Auntie Maggie and Nurse Glenys. They brought warmth to the ward. They were surrogate mothers. I can understand the younger children suffering from post-traumatic stress disorder because children need to be nurtured so they can develop properly. Auntie Maggie would bring in a catalogue at Christmas and tell us to save our money to choose a present for our parents. During the week the food was not that great. I remember a Sunday they had turkey and stuffing, which I love. I must have put on twenty pounds when I was there because I loved the Sunday dinners. The balcony seemed like a separate community. Someone had washed my twin-set and it was so cold that it had frozen stiff and fallen down the balcony rails. Everybody laughed. Then I was moved to the Six-Bedder. I remember we had torches. We were in the Girl Guides and we used to do the Morse on the ceiling. I taught a girl called Ann how to do the Morse. At the tail end of the treatment I spent a lot of time with Edgar the gardener, the dog (Paddy), Lady the horse, and the swans (Peter and Wendy).

I don't have bad memories but whenever I went for an X-ray I worried myself into a state. I used to think, 'I don't feel sick,' so I had no indication that I was getting better. It gave me a full appreciation of medicine and I think is one of the reasons I went into the medical profession. I have been in the States for about forty-five years. I came to the University of Chicago to study. I was already a midwife. The history of Craig-y-nos goes along with the history of TB. It does not have the stigma that it did years ago. If we as patients can talk about it that could be a precedent of the book.

Marlene met her husband in California and has been married for forty-three years. She has four children and five grandchildren and is an American citizen.

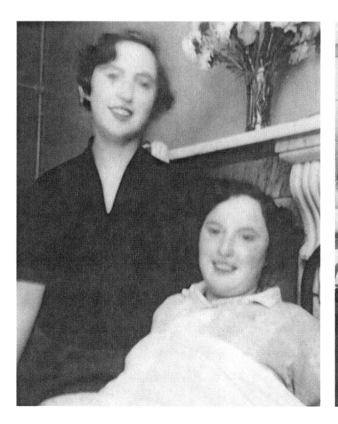
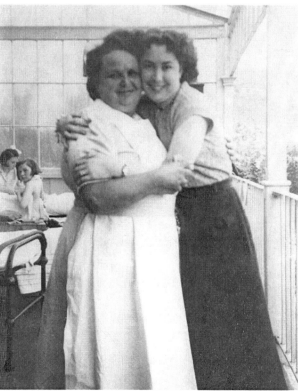

Marian Thomas (John) – Thomas plays ghost

'Why has Mr Williams got tears in his eyes?' I remember thinking as the ambulance driver, who was our neighbour, drove me to Craig-y-nos. He knew, but I didn't, that I was going to be in for a very long time. It was 1953 and I was fifteen. I was put in Ward 2. I asked the girl in the next bed how long she had been in and she said, 'Six years.' I sobbed and sobbed at nights for months.

I had not been there long before they talked about Adelina Patti appearing at a certain time in the night. Well, one evening the piano started playing. It scared me stiff. We think someone had put Sister Morgan's cat (Thomas) on it. It used to come into the ward from time to time. Nobody ever owned up. There was an occasion when we had nothing but potatoes and gravy for dinner. We kept asking 'Where's the meat?' Auntie Maggie felt sorry for us and brought us in some chips one day, and would you believe it, we had chips for supper that night! On the whole, I have happy memories of the place apart from feeling very cold with the only heating being hot water bottles. I took six O-Levels while I was there but the school authorities claimed the exams had not been properly invigilated and so they were not awarded. I was so disappointed. All my books and satchel were taken away to be decontaminated but I never saw them again.

On leaving Craig-y-nos in 1955, I remember crying in the car and my father smiling and asking me if I wanted to go back. I didn't, but just felt sad that I was leaving all my friends behind. Even though I had my own bedroom at home with a big bay window, I still felt lonely and it felt so small after the castle. I worked as an auxiliary nurse for more than twenty years. I think having had the experience of Craig-y-nos, it makes you a more caring person. I realize, looking back, that there was no psychological or emotional support for the children.

Marian is married with a son and grandson.

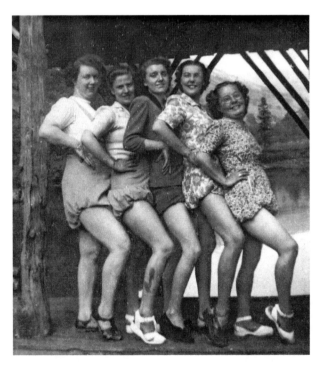

Show a leg! Marian and friends cut loose at the boat house. Courtesy Marian Thomas.

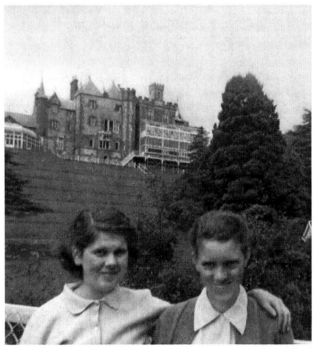

Sandra and Christine stand on the bridge over the River Tawe with the backdrop of the Castle towering above. Courtesy Christine Perry.

Margaret Blake (Howells) – Wilfred Pickles and the chocolate bars

I lived in a remote hill farm, Ty-Groes, under the Table Mountain, high above Llanbedr village, near Crickhowell, on the edge of the Black Mountains. The farm had no electricity. We had nothing to do in the evenings except sit around the kitchen table, and talk. They would tell stories of how TB had wiped out whole families in the area. Well, I got pleurisy in 1953 and I was in Crickhowell Hospital for a time, then I got moved to Craig-y-nos. I asked the girls what was wrong with them and each one said 'TB', and I said 'I've got pleurisy.' The girls said, 'No, you haven't. You've got TB like the rest of us.' Well, I cried and cried for weeks because I thought I was going to die, but streptomycin had arrived. Once I realized I was not going to die, I enjoyed myself at Craig-y-nos. I am gregarious by nature and I loved the company. Craig-y-nos brought me out. It gave me self-confidence.

One summer, I helped the gardeners pick caterpillars off the cabbages. We used to have Girl Guides with singsongs around a 'pretend' fire in the middle of Ward 2. I remember the radio entertainer, Wilfred Pickles. One day he broadcast a wish to give every child in Craig-y-nos a bar of chocolate. Well, the next thing we know, boxes and boxes of chocolate start arriving! We had chocolate we had never seen before. Dr Hubbard was a nasty bit of work. One day, she announced which girls were allowed to put curlers in their hair and which were not allowed. She said I could have curlers, but the other girls wouldn't let me. They said if they couldn't have curlers then neither could I.

I was so excited when it came time for me to go home but it was an anticlimax. I missed the company. I was fourteen so I went back to the local secondary modern school until I was fifteen. I wasn't much good at school because I had lost such a lot of education.

Margaret became a nanny. Today, she is married with three daughters and six grandsons.

Pass the test

Craig-y-nos towers high above us
Holding memories of the past,
Such as Madame Patti singing
With a glorious voice that lasts.
With its walls so firmly standing
And a turret of the best,
It will guard us, be our refuge
Till at last we pass the test.

Margaret Blake (Howells)

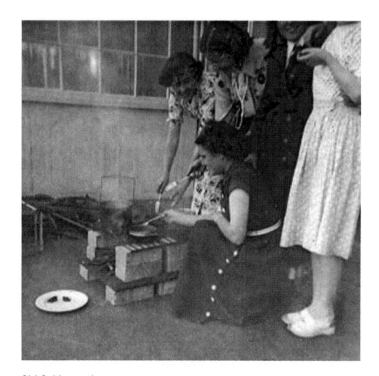

Girl Guides on the balcony of ward 2 light a real fire but what are they cooking? Courtesy Ann Shaw.

Sylvia Moore (Peckham) – Patient then nurse

I lived with my father and I think my TB was due, actually, to poor upbringing. I had appendicitis aged thirteen (1953) and was admitted to hospital where they discovered I had TB in both lungs. I was really poorly and for the first eighteen months in Craig-y-nos I was in a room on my own, lying on my back. When I was admitted I remember Dr Hubbard saying to me, 'Do you like milk?' And I said, 'Yes, yes.' I was almost too frightened to talk to her. She said, 'Good. You drink for me lots of milk - four or five pints a day - and we'll get on well together.' A very formidable lady but she had the patients' interests at heart. After eighteen months, I was joined by Theresa Thomas (O'Leary). She was another one who wasn't expected to go out and we became great friends. Later, I was moved onto Ward 2 balcony.

I received no schooling because I was so ill. I'm self-taught. I remained flat on my back for three years, not allowed to write or do anything. I had streptomycin during all that time. One year, we'd had this television set donated, and I asked if I could watch Wimbledon (the tennis tournament), which I adored. Nurse Glenys Davies said, 'If you sit up, I shall put the screens around you for the rest of the day.' I was feeling so sorry for myself but after about twenty minutes, in she comes with two porters dragging an enormous dressing table with a mirror on it, which they positioned so that I could watch Wimbledon. Craiy-y-nos was our home, a wonderful place. We had a great deal of fun there. I used to roll bottles across the ward in the middle of the night. Other children thought it was ghosts and were petrified. In the evenings, when Matron Knox-Thomas came on her six o'clock round, she'd be accompanied by her beautiful red setter dog, Paddy. The nurses had to roll down their sleeves and put their white cuffs on, and stand by the beds. Sister (Betty) Lewis (who was appointed following the retirement of Sister Winnie Morgan) was lovely but wasn't very good at controlling us. We were misbehaving one day and she came into the ward with a bandage around her head, which she had smeared with jam. She said, 'Look what you have done. You've made Sister bang her head. Now, will you all please be quiet.' Dr Patrick Mulhall did his very first bronchoscopy on me. When I met him again in 2007, he said, 'Oh my word, you survived!'

I was discharged as a patient in November 1957, along with Theresa O'Leary and Diane Hughes. Dr Williams (the Medical Superintendent) got us together and said, 'Don't you think it would be a wonderful idea if you came back to nurse here?' We all looked at each other and thought, 'Well, great,' because that's an offer of a job, isn't it? Of course, it was a ploy to keep an eye on us. I was there for about two and a half years, towards the end of which I met my husband, Donald, who had just started work as an engineer at Craig-y-nos. One day he was walking past the nurses' home, and for devilment, I squirted him with water. We married ten months later. When I was twenty-four, I became seriously ill with aspergillosis (a severe lung infection caused by a fungus of the *Aspergillus* species). It had obviously got into a lung cavity that I still had from the TB. I was haemorrhaging rather badly and I went into the Brompton Hospital, London. A Professor (Guy) Scadding diagnosed it and I had virtually the entire left lung removed. Afterwards, the very first thing they said to me was, 'What you need to do is to go and get yourself pregnant.' That's exactly what I did. I had two children, a boy and a girl.

Sylvia and her husband live in Talgarth (Powys).

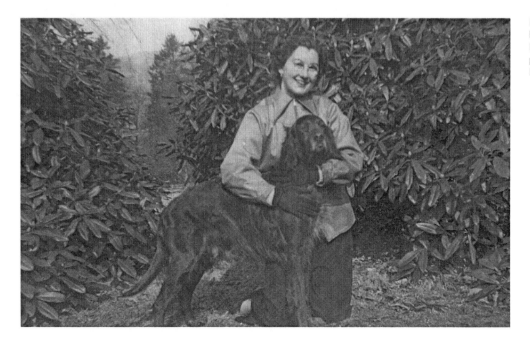

Paddy, the Irish Setter belonging to Matron Knox-Thomas, with a patient, Jean. Courtesy Mary Watkins.

Pass the test

Craig-y-nos towers high above us
Holding memories of the past,
Such as Madame Patti singing
With a glorious voice that lasts.
With its walls so firmly standing
And a turret of the best,
It will guard us, be our refuge
Till at last we pass the test.

Margaret Blake (Howells)

Myfanwy Blatchford (Hoyles) – The premonition

My father's brother died in Craig-y-nos as the clock struck midnight. When it was my turn to go there in 1953, this was in my mind, and every night I was fighting to stay awake until that clock had struck midnight. And then I could sleep. The only treatment I received was fresh air, food and rest. I was in bed for a month and then I was up and about playing havoc! Everybody was friends.

One day Mari Friend (Jenkins) and I took a little boat out on the lake. We couldn't get back and Alfie Repado, the gardener, had to come and rescue us. We were confined to bed as a punishment. Dr Hubbard used to frighten me. She was strange looking - rather manly, and her accent too. She gave me heck because I had a vest on (my mother made sure I had vests to wear under my pyjamas because I was sleeping outside). 'Take zat off! Vot eeze zat you got on! You muz let your body breathe.' She made me strip it all off. My brother's wife, who had been in a sanatorium up north for seven years, was transferred to Craig-y-nos. My family was allowed to visit her every week so I could at least wave to them through the window. After visiting, we would go halfway down the stairs and there would be a parcel of food left there for us. We used to go up on the roof for a midnight feast – wonderful. I remember our ward teas - the big enamel trays stacked high with bread and butter, a bottle of red sauce and a bottle of brown sauce. We were starving after being out all day.

Something very strange happened one night. We had been to the Patti theatre. It was a wild night on the balcony - windy and cold. We had tied the tarpaulins on our beds and I woke up during the night, and the canvas on my bed was rising. I was terrified. I could see Caroline, the little girl from the next bed, standing looking at me. Caroline had never walked in her life. I panicked and rang my bell. Nobody came. I went under the bed clothes and stayed there. The following day the specialist came and said that Caroline was to get calipers for her legs. It was like a premonition, very frightening. Craig-y-nos did me a lot of good because, at fourteen, I was very shy. It was the company and seeing people worse off than yourself. I wanted to work with flowers but they wouldn't let me because of the pollen, so they put me into Gorseinon Technical College to do a secretarial course.

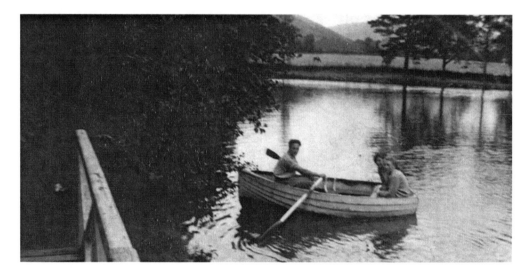

Myfanwy and Mari being rescued by Alfie the gardener after taking a rowing boat onto the lake. Courtesy Myfanwy Blatchford.

Mary Ireland (Jones) – Bad news

My periods started on my first night in Craig-y-nos in 1950. I asked Dorothy, in the next bed, if she had a towel. She rummaged in her locker and found me one. Next morning, Dorothy got a row for making a noise in the night, so I explained that it was my fault. I was put to lie on my right side for eight months but never had any drugs during the two years I was there.

We lived in Llangattock, just outside Crickhowell, and the round trip was over seventy miles. Transport was very difficult in those days. I don't know how my mother would have managed if Mrs Rumsey, the mother of a timid, shy little girl call Ann (Shaw), hadn't given her a lift on visiting days. One visiting day, Dr Hubbard called my mother into the office and told her that unless I had a lobectomy (removal of part of a lung), I would die, and they were sending me home to wait for a place at Sully Hospital, Cardiff. Well, my mother was terribly upset, so some of the other parents took her to the local pub for a drink! I was sent home but by the time a vacancy came up at Sully, they decided I was cured and didn't need the operation after all.

I was sixteen when I left Craig-y-nos and had lost out on my education. I went to work in a chemist's shop in Abergavenny.

Mary has been married for fifty years and lives in Gloucestershire. She has four children and five grandchildren.

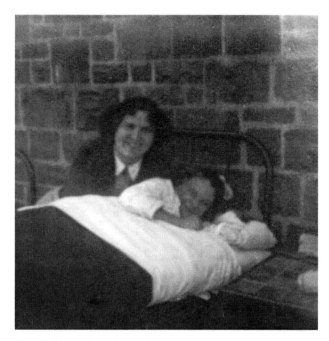

Mary (left) with Ann Shaw, whose
mother used to give Mary's mother
a lift to Craig-y-nos on visiting days.
Courtesy Ann Shaw.

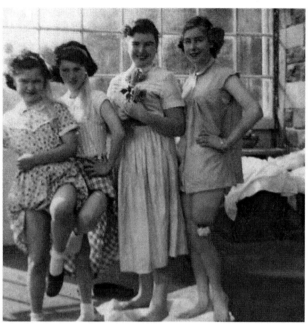

Balcony dancers. Christine is second
left. With the coming of successful
drug treatment for TB, the atmosphere
amongst patients in the 1950s was more
positive than in previous decades.
Courtesy Christine Perry.

Christine Perry (Bennett) – Fireworks

I went into Craig-y-nos two days before my thirteenth birthday in 1954 and came out two weeks before my sixteenth birthday. It was one of the happiest times of my life. The place was full when I went in but not many people were left there by 1957. I've revisited Ward 2 recently, and I reckon that it held about twenty beds. It seems hard to believe in such a confined space but the beds must have been small and close together.

To while away the time we entertained ourselves with activities such as 'ad hoc' singing competitions - Eisteddfodau, you could call them, I suppose! 'Ave, Maria' I considered to be my party piece but I flannelled my way through it as I didn't know all of the Latin (some ex-patients recall Christine entertaining the ward with her beautiful singing voice). We were also good at play-acting and mimicry. Dr Hubbard was obviously a prime candidate. Two of us managed to 'borrow' Dr Hubbard's white coat from her lounge on her day off. We both got into the very large coat, one behind the other, in order to replicate her rather large behind. We then had to walk, as she did, dragging one foot, from her lounge into the ward. We should have got an Oscar for that! We had a Girl Guides group, and I was so enthusiastic about guiding activities, that I was promoted to Leader. Three of us escorted the Standard to Abercrave Church (where it remains today) so that it could be blessed. Dr Williams, the Medical Superintendent, and his wife took us in their car. This was the first time I had been outside the hospital grounds in two years. We had a lovely day but shortly afterwards I suffered my third relapse and had to return to bed.

We weren't allowed onto the roof of the castle or beyond the bridge over the river but we did both. In summer, we could ford the river without being seen from the hospital. Then we could move up through the woods to the lake to see the swans or ride the horses belonging to Dr Williams' daughters. I remember Joan, the young deaf girl, who was a travellers' child. Miss White, the teacher, brought in a sign language book for us to teach ourselves, which the older girls did without exception. Joan's mother didn't visit too regularly. It seemed to us that she didn't care much about Joan's predicament. When patients' teatime came around, her mother would eat Joan's tea and Joan wouldn't complain. It was clear that Joan wouldn't get Christmas presents so, along with the staff, we all contributed from our own gifts so that she didn't feel left out on Christmas morning. Bonfire night was also celebrated. Parents were allowed to bring in fireworks beforehand and the gardeners would make up a bonfire in the grounds where it could be viewed from the balcony. A girl named Rita managed to secrete a few sparklers and matches, which were produced after lights out. She dished these out amongst us and we proceeded to light up! Immediately, the call went up, 'Nurse coming!' The sparklers were doused and hidden in lockers but Rita decided to keep hers going under the bedclothes. 'What's that smoke and what's that smell of burning?' At which point, Rita's bed began to get hot and she started to panic 'Oh, OOOH!!' She had burnt her sheets and had to spend a few hours with her bed pulled out into the corridor - a pretty standard form of punishment.

Dr Hubbard terrified me. We had monthly examinations in her office and she always used to complain, 'This child never puts on any weight.' When I was leaving Craig-y-nos, my grandmother, who had brought me up, went to thank her and Dr Huppert shouted, 'Don't thank me. If I had my way she would be in for another year until she had put on some weight!' I weighed six stones (38.18 kgs) then and I still weigh the same. Adjusting to life at home was very difficult. My Gran couldn't understand why I was not pleased to be home. I was an only child. In Craig-y-nos I had lots of company. At home the house seemed so small and the ceilings so low. Also, I had left school and it was another year before I was allowed to start work.

My husband and I celebrated our Ruby wedding in 2007 by going back to Craig-y-nos Castle and spending the night in the bridal suite, the former private chapel of Adelina Patti.

Christine has three sons and one grandchild.

May Bennett (Snell) - The visiting tortoise

I remember the excitement one Saturday morning in 1956 when Dr Hubbard announced, 'From now on, you've all got visiting every weekend.' Until then, only patients over the age of sixteen had weekly visitors. I immediately wrote a letter to my parents, which was delivered to them in Penclawdd by the fiancé of a patient in Ward 4: 'If you can, come up tomorrow. Just jump on the bus.' My aunt and uncle came as well because Nurse Meikel had told them. It was a close community. Astrid's mum brought a tortoise for her to see, and my uncle wrote it up for the local paper: 'George, the tortoise comes to visit'. Dr Hubbard went on the rampage and demanded to know who had done it. She said, 'Nobody's going to have visitors until we know.' I said, 'I think it's my uncle that's done this.' He had to go and see her the next weekend. Dr Hubbard inspired fear, not only among the children, but their parents too.

Two of the girls were confirmed in the Patti theatre, which was a big thing, and I went to watch. We weren't allowed upstairs to visit the little ones and neither were we allowed into the 'Six Bedder', where the older girls were, but friendships did develop. We used to go for X-rays and I met Mary Cullen from Swansea. Mary started sending me little cakes, with a note saying, 'From your X-ray pal, Mary.' I've got a photograph of Mary that she gave me, and on the back it says, 'From your X-ray pal.' Years ago people would say, 'You go to Craig-y-nos and you don't come out.' But I was there in the fifties and I had streptomycin. Nevertheless, I was very slight and Dr Hubbard said, 'Oh, you can't go home. You've got to put weight on.' So I put fruit in the pockets of my dressing gown before I was weighed, but they sussed that out.

I found it a strange going back to a small terraced house after living in a castle. I missed the company and the routine. I was fourteen and I never went back to grammar school because I was told it would be too stressful. Instead, I went to Gorseinon Technical College and became a shorthand typist. Before I got married I asked if it would be alright to have children and they said, 'Yes, it's fine.'

May has two children and four grandchildren.

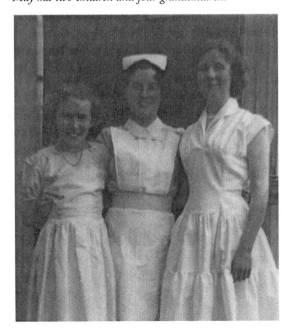

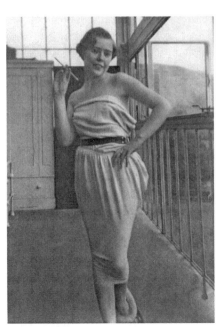

Pat Curry (left) and Ann Davies in their confirmation frocks. They were confirmed in the Patti Theatre. Nurse May Jones is centre. Courtesy Christine Perry.

May in model pose and fluffy slippers, but what *is* she wearing? Courtesy May Bennett.

Mair Harris (Edwards) – Lost teenage years

Craig-y-nos made me independent. Staff could take your parents' place to a certain extent but otherwise you had to do everything on your own. I was admitted as a thirteen-year-old in 1950 and spent most of my twenty-two months there on the balcony of Ward 2. I have very positive memories and made lots of friends. I learned how to write letters and had many pen pals. There were no phones. Once you were up for two or four hours you would be allowed to dress. Christmas was fantastic! I used to go to the Patti theatre and there would be Santa Claus (Jenkyn Evans, the hospital dentist) and presents from the Friends of the hospital. I remember having a huge jigsaw. We were allowed to put up pillow cases that were filled with parcels from home. I remember having seventy or eighty presents!

Miss White, the teacher, told me to send for my school books and helped me so much that when I went back to grammar school I had not fallen far behind. Unfortunately, I had two relapses and was back in sanatoriums. I was nineteen before I was better so I missed out on my teenage years. I was going to go in for teaching but I couldn't because I had had TB. My mother felt it best that I stayed at home rather than go away to college so I worked in the library. I was an assistant librarian throughout my career. I come back to Craig-y-nos for the summer sometimes, to walk around the lake like I used to.

Mary Watkins (Williams) – Streptomycin's miracle

I was close to death when I was admitted to Craig-y-nos in 1955. According to Nurse Glenys Davies, I wasn't expected to live more than a fortnight, but I was started on streptomycin and, miraculously, began to recover. At first though, I was isolated in an attic room before being moved to Sister Morgan's office. I had TB in both lungs and for thirteen months lay immobile in a plaster cast on my left side. Eventually, I was moved into Ward 2 and then onto the balcony.

Lying so still, I would hear the lift gates clanking open and Dr Hubbard shouting if she heard anyone talking. 'Pull zat girl out into ze corridor!' and beds would be pulled out. Once I was better and allowed up, I have pleasant memories of my stay. Indeed, I would not be here today but for Craig-y-nos. I was transferred to Sully Hospital, Cardiff, for a lung operation before finally being discharged at the age of sixteen and a half. Home was very strange at first. It was so quiet and I missed the company. However, at seventeen, I got my driving licence and an open-air job – driving a bakery van around the Brecon and Talgarth countryside. I did this for eight years before getting married and moving to Hereford. In September 2007, I was reunited with Glenys Davies after more than fifty years.

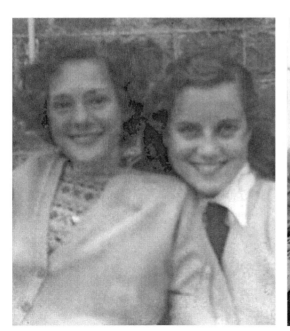 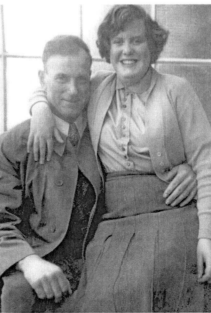

Mair (right) with her friend Shirley. Courtesy Ann Shaw.

Mary with her father on Ward 2 balcony. Her life was saved by streptomycin. Courtesy Mary Watkins.

Ann Peters (Williams) – The bird tamer

I was known as 'Ann on blocks' because the foot of my bed was raised on twelve-inch blocks to stop my lung haemorrhages. My father died of TB when I was about five and my two sisters and a brother had also been ill. My father's sister was in Craig-y-nos at the same time as me but, unfortunately, she died too. I was just over eleven when I was admitted in 1954 and was flat on my back for sixteen months, on streptomycin and PAS (para-aminosalicylic acid). Dr Hubbard told my mother that it would be twelve months before they'd know if I was 'out of the woods'. Dr Hubbard was a lovely person. It's just that she was so very abrupt, but she was nice to me. I never felt ill. I used to think, 'Why on earth am I here?' I don't think any of the girls really felt ill although I do remember Mary Watkins (Williams). She had a terrible, terrible cough. Every morning they would bring her over the bed and thump her back to get rid of what was on her chest.

Even though I couldn't sit up, they'd position me where I could watch the telly, and the girls would all come around to talk to me. I could see who was coming in and out of the ward with a hand mirror. From my bed on the balcony, I would entice robins and sparrows to sit on my hand by holding out crumbs of bread. Life on the balcony was cold but at the time, it didn't seem as if there was anything wrong or hard about it. We were all in the same position and nobody complained. Someone bought me a typewriter and I learned to do shorthand out of a 'Teach Yourself' book. When I was allowed to get dressed, some of us bought bright orange trousers. I don't know why - we could be seen for miles. The grounds were lovely. We also used to go down to the basement where they kept 'Jimmy the skeleton' (for training the nurses). One of the girls would blow into an empty bottle, making an eerie noise, and we'd frighten the new girls.

Today, I have restricted mobility. I've had both hips replaced and have been on sticks for four years. One leg is two inches shorter than the other and is painful all the time, but it's now part of me and doesn't stop me getting where I want to go.

Ann has four children and three grandchildren.

Norma Lewis (Pearce) – First kiss

Harry Secombe gave me my first kiss. I went to see him in the Christmas pantomime in the Patti theatre (1953) and he came around the ward afterwards and kissed everyone. I was thirteen. At eleven, my father had died of TB in Sully Hospital, Cardiff, after being there for three years. I now realize what a hard time my mother had. She used to bring me a parcel of food every Saturday morning and we'd have midnight feasts on the balcony. I remember the tarpaulins on the bed and how we had to be kept cold. When you think about it now, it was crazy.

The young women in the 'Six Bedder' befriended us. Pat Hybert (Mogridge), who was about twenty, used to write letters and send me sweets and bars of chocolate although she wasn't allowed to come into the ward to see me. I kept in contact with her for quite a while. I have no bad recollections, really, of my time there. It did affect me in some ways. I am very independent and quite like my own company, much as I like other people. I was astonished to discover that Rosie Pugh (Hunt), whom I have known for over thirty years, had also been in Craig-y-nos. It was something of our past we had never talked about until I saw pictures of her in the photographic exhibition.

Even though I had drug treatment, I came out of Craig-y-nos worse than when I went in. Mum took me to Grove Place Chest Clinic, Swansea, and I had a lung removed the day after my fifteenth birthday (1955), in Cimla Hospital, Neath, where I remained for six months. On one occasion it was snowing and there were no buses, so my mother walked all the way to the hospital to see me. It must have been a distance of some fifteen miles.

Opposite page

The bird tamer. Ann entices wild birds onto her hand with crumbs of bread. Courtesy Beryl Richards.

Frozen landscape. Even the swan is standing on ice. Cold air was considered beneficial for tuberculosis and children were outdoors as much as possible. Courtesy Christine Perry.

Temperature chart of a girl with tuberculosis of the lungs. Her temperature over one month is continually and rapidly rising and falling (from 103.2° F (40° C) to 97.3° F (36° C) as her body tries to fight the infection. Wellcome Images, London.

The TB flushes

Norma Lewis (Pearce) remembers Auntie Maggie and Nurse Glenys Davies tucking them in at night in Ward 2 and singing *The TB Flushes*.

I have the TB flushes,	The van was very rocky,	'Mama, Dada fetch me out
I have them very bad.	It nearly knocked me out	From this isolation home.
They wrapped me up in blankets	And when the door was opened	I have been here a year or two
And put me in the van,	I gave a mighty shout:	And now I want to be with you.'

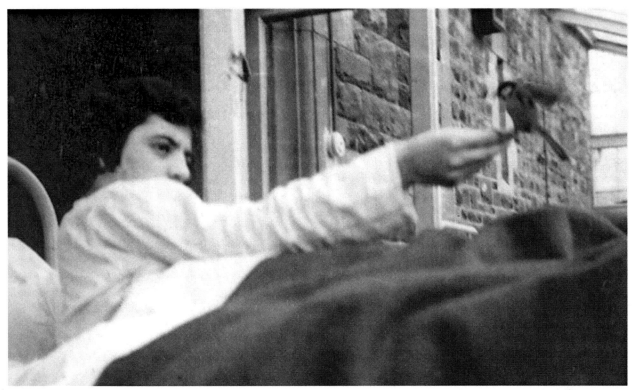

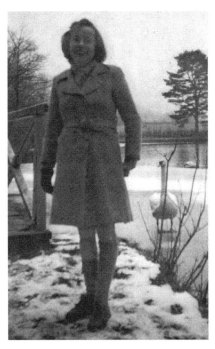

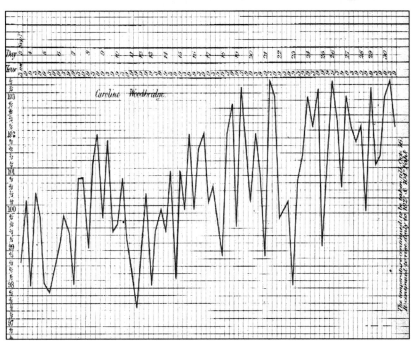

Delphine Barnes (Watkins) – Plaster bed

I remember receiving the letter to go into Craig-y-nos on my fifteenth birthday, and I was admitted two days later. It was 1951. At that time it was reckoned that if you went to Craig-y-nos you wouldn't come out alive. I went from a very loving family to this austere castle, and wasn't allowed visitors for five weeks. Nurse Davies was from Fforestfach, where I lived, and she looked after me as I was very homesick.

There was a rumour that Madame Patti haunted the wards, so you can imagine how scared I was, never having been away from home. They put me next to Shirley Osborne on the balcony. She was on a plaster bed, and little did I think that four years later I would be back in hospital with TB of the spine, lying on a plaster bed. Although Craig-y-nos was rather a grim place, you seem to only remember the comradeship of the girls you were with. Streptomycin had not been out very long, and PAS always made me sick. As for how long I was there, I can't remember - maybe a year. Later, when I was in Cardiff, with TB spine, the doctor told me that it would have taken far longer to get well if strep didn't suit me.

Barbara O'Connell (Paines) – Norman Wisdom's escape plan

It was the third anniversary of my husband's death when I made contact with 'The Children of Craig-y-nos'. I had been to his grave and my daughter said, 'Come and stay with us for a few hours.' She showed me the Internet and asked me to suggest something. I don't know why but I said, 'Adelina Patti Hospital'. Nothing came up. I said, 'Try Craig-y-nos?' And up popped Ann's blog! I couldn't believe it! So many memories came flooding back and I recognized many of the girls. I was in Craig-y-nos for a year (1952-53). I did get used to being there, but you had to. My three older sisters were in a sanatorium in Denbigh, North Wales, and my youngest sister had been ill with TB meningitis so my mother really had her share of worries. I remember when Norman Wisdom came to the hospital and told us how to escape by tying the sheets together and getting over the wall.

We did have nice food. I can remember waiting for Wednesday because we had rabbit stew. I also liked chocolate mousse. Eggs were boiled for so long that the inside was black and the yolk all dried up. To this day I cannot stand the smell of them. We had pilchards for breakfast, which I thought was unusual but got used to it. We had more time to ourselves once we were allowed into the grounds but we had to make sure we had our meals. We used to help the gardeners, Edgar and Alfie, put the hay on the back of the trailer, and have a ride. That was the best part of my stay in hospital. I didn't have many clothes as I had been in bed for over a year at home before I was admitted to Craig-y-nos, so one of the girls altered a pleated skirt and I ended up with a little wardrobe so that I could go out with the girls. We also went to a little shop down in the basement where you could buy stationery and toiletries. I had a gastric lavage every month and that was the most terrifying thing that ever happened to me.

We all sat around a small black and white television to watch the Coronation, and received a certificate and a mug and coin that I still have. One night, a few of us were messing around after lights out. I was by Rose Ryan's bed when we heard Matron coming. I got into Rose's bed and was so frightened that I wet in her bed. She got into trouble the next morning but she didn't say it was me because we would have all been in for it. Quite often, when we heard Dr Hubbard in the lift upstairs we would open our lift door so that she couldn't come down. My bed was by the locker where the school bags were kept, so I had the job of handing them out to the girls. They were green bags with ties on and your name. One morning, I got the bags and they fell to the floor. Miss White, the teacher, was shouting at me so I started throwing them off the balcony. I think three of us were sent downstairs to retrieve them.

The day I came home was a bad experience. I walked through the door and ducked down. It seemed as if the ceiling was on top of me, it was so claustrophobic. School friends didn't want to know me because I'd had TB. I saw my best friend coming out of a shop, spoke to her and she ignored me. I started work when I was sixteen, and eventually found a job in a polish factory that suited me. If I had a bad day the bosses would give me the easy jobs. I got married when I was twenty-one, and had a daughter. My second daughter was a blue baby (Barbara's children were 'rhesus' babies) and had to have her blood changed. My first son died at birth and two more sons were also blue. They were all given the BCG jab at birth. TB stayed with us. My sister's first daughter died of TB meningitis when she was four-years-old and my sister was taken into Sully Hospital, Cardiff, with her two young boys. My youngest daughter had TB aged nine, and my mother got it in old age. I am still not free of hospitals as I have osteoporosis, so I go for regular infusions and scans. But you carry on and don't give in. We have all had to fight otherwise we wouldn't be here to tell our stories.

On 5 June 2008, Barbara returned to Craig-y-nos for the first time after fifty-five years.

Joan Wotton (Thomas) – Sexual abuse

I was fifteen when I became a patient at Craig-y-nos in 1950, and like many others my time there was one of unhappiness. Dr Hubbard shouted at me for wearing a lilac bed jacket and Miss White (the teacher) told her not to be cross with me. I loved to sew and used to sing for the girls in the ward. One girl, Mary Ireland (Jones) knocked out my four front teeth. It was an accident though – she pulled the sheet from under me while I sat on a bedpan! I remember the dentist. He sort of sexually abused me. He fondled me and pressed himself up against me while I sat in the dentist chair. I never told a soul. I had toothache after that but I would not go back.

Two girls, Rita and Marjorie, ran away. They just walked out with the weekend visitors. They got as far as Ystradgynlais before being caught and brought back. My mother used to send me a comic – *Girl*, I think it was. It used to feature different areas of the country and I wrote asking them to come to Craig-y-nos. The editors wrote to the hospital authorities asking permission and I got in terrible trouble because of it.

How could they treat children the way they did without any thought or feeling? I am in my seventies but the trauma of those times still has a profound effect on me.

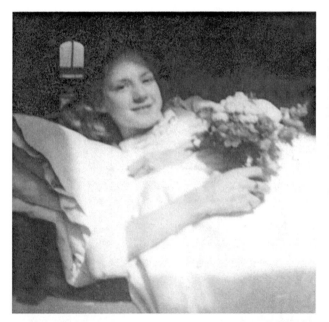 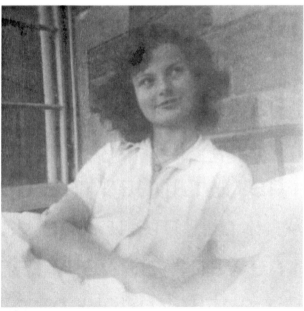

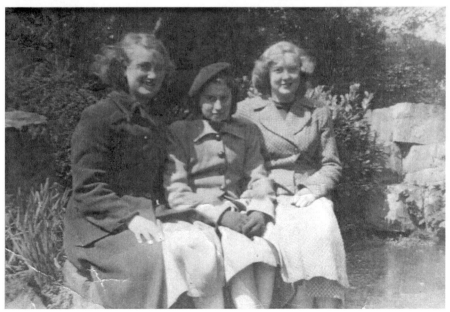

Shirley Osborne is lying on a plaster bed moulded to encase her body. She has tuberculosis of the spine. Courtesy Mari Friend.

Joan on the balcony of Ward 2. Courtesy Mari Friend.

Barbara (centre) with friends, Jean Griffiths (left) and Jean Shakeshaft. Barbara's four sisters also had TB. Courtesy Barbara O'Connell.

The TB flushes

I have the TB flushes,
I have them very bad.
They wrapped me up in blankets
And put me in the van,
The van was very rocky,
It nearly knocked me out
And when the door was opened
I gave a mighty shout:
'Mama, Dada fetch me out
From this isolation home.
I have been here a year or two
And now I want to be with you.'

Norma Lewis (Pearce)

Young women's stories

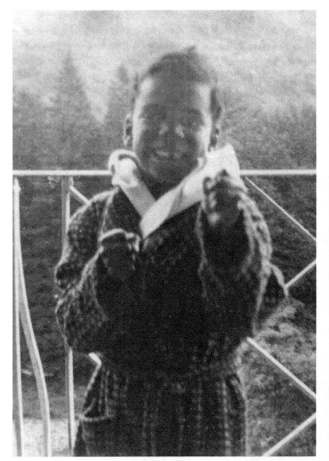

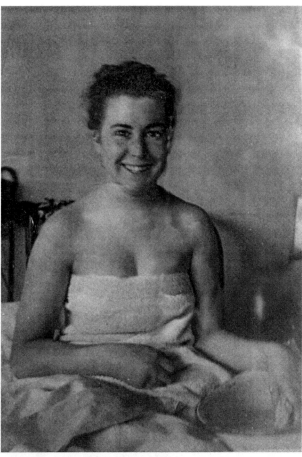

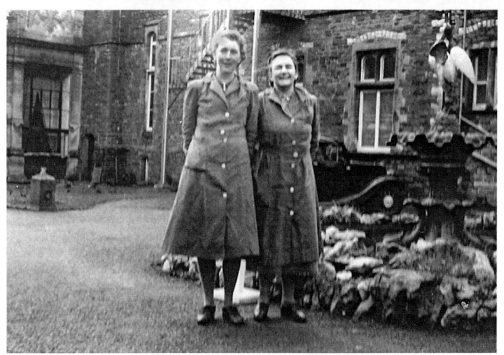

Robert Spetti, a balcony boy mimics the stance of 1952 British and Empire Heavyweight Champion, Welsh-born, Johnny Williams. Courtesy Sylvia Cottle.

Molly had this photograph taken for her husband and added the caption, 'Would you please washmy back darling?' Courtesy Molly Barry.

Mrs Thomas (left) and Miss White, teachers at Craig-y-nos. Courtesy Mary Ireland.

Eileen Gibbons (Hill) - Runaway

I used to sit and watch visitors leave through the courtyard. One Saturday, I walked out with them, had a glass of pop in the pub where the Brecon bus picked up passengers, and went home to Hay-on-Wye. It was a stupid thing to do but I'd lost my father only a few months before going into Craig-y-nos (1951) and I was very close to him. He was only fifty-four.

I was nineteen and a student nurse at Bronllys hospital, near Talgarth (Powys), when I caught TB. I was very lucky because streptomycin had been just discovered but it had a very bad effect on me. I had a fever and was very ill for about two months. Being young, I never thought about dying. It was months before I had my long hair washed. The nurse used to clean it with eau de cologne. I was in a room with three beds and on the balcony outside were children. There were grids in the floor and we used to get visitors (rats) sometimes running up and down! My family would bring me eggs and farm butter but you had to be careful because of the rats. I did tapestry when I was allowed to, and I had lots and lots of pen friends. You just passed the time.

After I'd run away, Dr Williams saw me at clinic in Brecon and went on treating me with help from my local doctor and nurse. He was a wonderful, *wonderful* man. I had a couple of relapses and more streptomycin. I got married but lost three little boys. In those days, after losing a child, you went straight back on the ward with the new mothers and you had to get on with it. I had my daughter after ten years but we were foster parents and that helped a lot.

Eileen lives in Herefordshire and has four grandchildren.

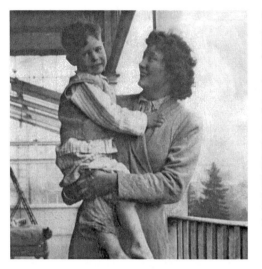 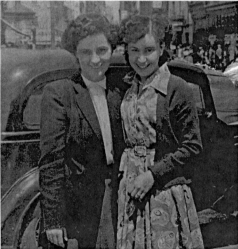

Eileen with a young boy on the balcony. Courtesy Eileen Gibbons.

Molly (right) in Swansea with Nurse 'Glen', after her discharge from Craig-y-nos. Courtesy Molly Barry.

The isolated location of Craig-y-nos contributed to its prison-like appearance. From a postcard, 1950s.

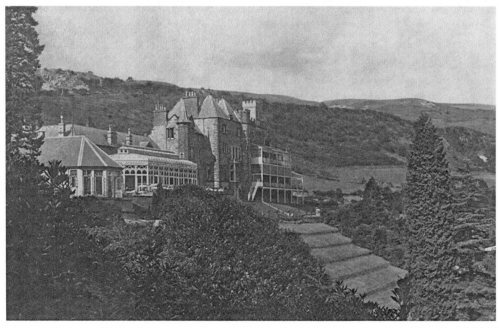

Euryl Thomas – Patient to secretary

Evil people said that my mother, Mrs Thomas, had carried the germ back from Craig-y-nos because she worked there as a teacher. The day I discovered I had TB, at the age of twenty (1950), my mother was teaching and Daddy was out and I hadn't worked for weeks. I got up but didn't feel like breakfast so I went back to bed. Our big black Persian cat crept up beside me and I started to cough. I felt the blood in my mouth and went down the stairs and it was pouring out of me.

They started me on streptomycin immediately and I had four injections a day. Dr Williams told my family that they couldn't promise anything but three weeks would tell whether the treatment was working or not. During that time no one was allowed to see me. There were twenty-six in the ward and four of my friends died in the six months I was there. I vividly recall Dilys Powell, in the next bed. She was so ill they could do nothing for her so she was going home. Nurse Davies took her in the ambulance but it couldn't get up to their remote farm so Dilys' father brought a 'gambo' (horse drawn wagon) to meet them. I don't think she lived a fortnight. I found it very upsetting and kept asking Dr Williams if I could go home. I even asked my own doctor and he sent me a card while he was on holiday, saying, 'Please try and settle down there for your own good.' I had a massive haemorrhage. My temperature went up and I thought I was coughing my lung up - it was like pennies – but it was the blood that I had swallowed. Streptomycin saved my life. I had it in 1950 and again in 1953. It took longer to cure the second time but I didn't go into hospital the second time.

Craig-y-nos felt like a prison. The regime was terrible. Eventually, you were allowed to do some embroidery and knitting but not for very long. We had 'silence hours' in the morning and afternoon where you just had to lie still. I was terribly unhappy and in the end Dr Williams said, 'We will allow you to go home as long as you don't get out of bed,' so my mother used to change the sheets with me still on the bed.

Having TB changed the course of my life. I was a sports girl and played tennis, and it all stopped even though I was cured. I had received voice training which I had to give up. I was told not to sing. Now I play the piano and I did have a small choir. I have always been attached to music. I went back to Craig-y-nos to work as the medical secretary for eighteen years. When the hospital closed, I was responsible for putting all the medical records on microfiche, and was later told that I should have been wearing a mask before opening the boxes (those records have since disappeared). However, I still have my own case notes. Dr Williams gave them to me when he left. They are written in Dr Hubbard's spidery writing. One note says that I was seriously ill with 'massive increase in disease in ten days.'

Molly Barry (O'Shea) – Ghostly encounters

I was in the Six-Bedder next to the big children's ward (Ward 2). One night, we heard the children shouting because they'd seen a figure in white. Sister Morgan accused me of scaring them but it wasn't me. Then the door to our ward, which was always propped open with a heavy stool, closed of its own accord. I was full of wickedness but I didn't do it.

I was admitted to Craig-y-nos in March 1950, celebrated my twenty-first birthday there (March 1951), was discharged in May, got married by special licence, and was re-admitted in December for another nine months. I had streptomycin and PAS (para-aminosalicylic acid) – huge white tablets that I couldn't swallow. They used to make me vomit. When I got a bit more 'with it', I would arrange the flowers, lying on my left side. I'd also write letters for other people and write my own letters every day, but otherwise just read. Every day a little robin used to come in and perch on the foot of my bed. Sometimes I'd be taken down in my bed to the Patti Theatre so see a concert or film show, which was lovely.

I had two children and am now a great grandmother. I worked as a nurse.

Every night, during the photographic exhibition of The Children of Craig-y-nos in Brecon Library, the picture of Molly, in a corner of the gallery, fell off the wall. The first task of the librarian each morning was to hang it up again. One morning it was at right-angles to the corner and upright; impossible for it to have landed in that position.

Olive Pamela Joseph - Thunderstorm

My husband's job in the quarry ended and we went to live on my parents'farm at Ynystawe, about five miles out of Swansea. I couldn't climb the stairs, I was so weak, but the doctor kept putting off an X-ray. Eventually, I said, 'If you don't take me to have an X-ray now, I'm going to get another doctor.' So, he took me to the local cottage hospital, and then came to tell me I had TB. I hadn't eaten for three months and weighed less than six stones (38.18 kgs). They started me on streptomycin and Rimifon (isoniazid, discovered in 1952). I went to Craig-y-nos in May 1956, just after my twenty-seventh birthday, and came home the following November, weighing fourteen stones (89.09 kgs)! I didn't get out of bed until three months before I came home and never saw my children (a girl aged six and a boy of four) all the time I was in there.

The nurses were marvellous but Dr Hubbard was horrible, really *horrible!* She said, 'This lady is here solely because she had all her teeth out.' She was making out that I hadn't been looking after myself. She'd say, 'Don't curl your hair. You're not supposed to lift your hands up.' But everybody wanted to make themselves a bit special. Oh dear, dear! I hated to see her coming round. I was on the balcony when we had a terrible thunderstorm. You could see the lightening striking the hill opposite and burning the grass. Matron Knox-Thomas, a lovely lady, came down in her dressing gown with her dog, and no teeth! She said, 'Make tea for these ladies, all of them, and if you haven't got enough, come upstairs to my flat and take what you want.'

The worst thing was not seeing my children but they were with my parents and had a good life. When I came out of Craig-y-nos, I had another child and had to have streptomycin all the way through the pregnancy. I went down to the clinic when I was carrying the fourth one and the doctor said, 'You're looking wonderful.' I said, 'I feel terrible having a baby again.' 'Go on,' she said, 'You've got a lovely family, and a healthy woman like you.' I had another one after that. Unfortunately, I lost my husband when I was forty-seven. He had a brain haemorrhage. So I had to bring the children up myself.

Olive has nineteen grandchildren and twelve great-grandchildren.

Pat Hybert (Mogridge) – Dracula and the dentist

I remember going to the dentist (Jenkyn Evans) at Craig-y-nos because I had a bad tooth. When I came back to the ward I thought, 'He hasn't taken the bad tooth. He's taken the next one, twit.' So I had two gaps and I had to wear false teeth. When my own dentist saw them, he said, 'I've never seen such awful false teeth.'

It was snowing in December 1952 when I was admitted to Craig-y-nos, aged nineteen. I'd had a lung haemorrhage three months earlier and the specialist came to the house straight away and put me on streptomycin and PAS (para-aminosalicylic acid). The streptomycin affected my hearing. I could feel my ears tingling. The doctors looked in my ears to see if they wanted syringing, but I don't think they were very interested, really. They were only interested in getting you cured. I'm completely deaf in one ear now and I later found out that it was a side effect of the antibiotic. It was a small price to pay, I suppose, for being fit and well again. Dr Williams was very nice but we used to call Dr Hubbard 'Dracula' because she'd come round doing loads of blood tests. They used to give us lots of milk, thinking that would do us good. Well, of course, we all put on a tremendous amount of weight. Even as adults, we were treated like school children. Harry Secombe did a panto at Christmas time, but I wasn't allowed to go because I'd got out of bed when I wasn't supposed to. Now, I wouldn't have taken it, but at the time you did as you were told. We were very naïve compared with today.

We did miss out on a lot of things in life. We couldn't go dancing and I was very wary of what I was doing afterwards. I was having check-ups for years. I returned to work in my office but discovered that two other people there had TB at the same time as me.

Pat has two children and three grandchildren.

Sylvia Cottle (Price) – The meaning of bed rest

I had started on streptomycin and bed rest at home but when I got into Craig-y-nos, in 1952, I found out what bed rest really meant! I had been there about a week when I leant out of bed to pick something up off the floor and got a *terrible* ticking off from the nurse followed by another from Dr Hubbard. My bed was on eighteen-inch blocks and I had to lie still in one position on my side. It's amazing what you can find to do even like that. I read and did embroidery.

They would bring a basin around every day for you to clean your teeth, but hair washing - I don't remember any in the year that I was there. We had a blanket bath once a week. One day, they took the blocks away and I felt as if I was sliding out of bed. It was a weird sensation. On my twenty-first birthday, my mother brought in a cold chicken. The girls in the ward bought me a Toby jug, which I still have. I shall always remember my fiancé sitting with snowflakes on his shoulder, blowing in through the windows, which of course, we were not allowed to close. You did as you were told and accepted things. People didn't protest like they do now. I also remember Robert Spetti, a little boy on the balcony, whose photograph I took.

I had a pneumothorax to collapse my lung but it didn't work so I was sent home to wait for a bed in Morriston Hospital. When I was eventually discharged, I had to wait a year before marrying but was told, 'No children for three years.' I went on to have four!

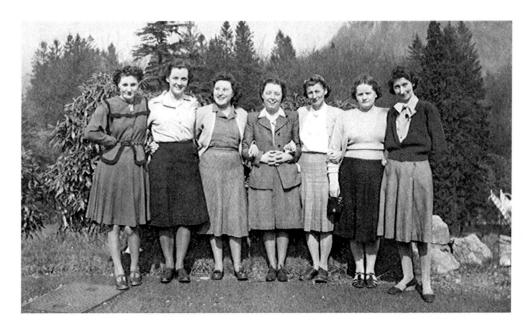

Young women in the Castle grounds. Many like Olive were married and spent months or years separated from their families. Courtesy Dulcie Oltersdorf.

Pat in the 'Six-Bedder', being careful not to show her teeth. Courtesy Pat Hybert.

Sylvia holding Bonzo the badger, one of the pets belonging to Dr Williams' daughters. Courtesy Sylvia Cottle.

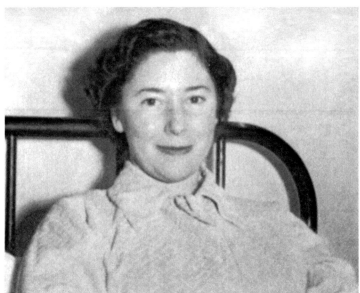

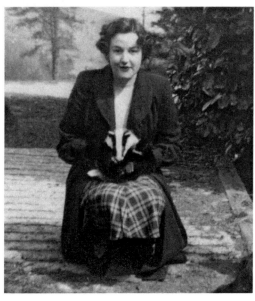

Relatives' stories

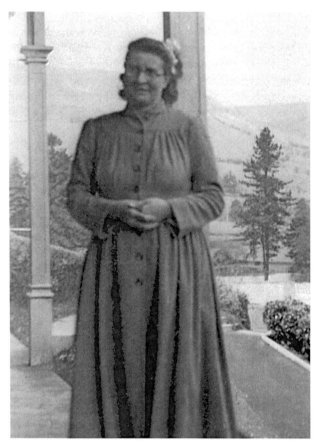

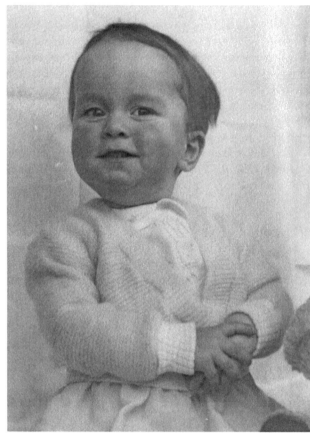

Ray beneath the
balcony block. Like
many patients on bed
rest and nourishing
food, she put on a
considerable amount
of weight. Courtesy
Ann Morris.

Christopher, a child with
cystic fibrosis. Courtesy
Peter Gunn.

Ann Morris – Mother's inflation

My mother, Rachel Lewis (known as 'Ray'), went into Craig-y-nos as a very thin, smart woman. Eighteen months later she came out weighing fifteen stone! She looked as if she had been inflated. I said, 'That's not my mother!' and burst out crying. Mother was very upset.

I was eight years of age and an only child when mother was admitted in 1951, but she'd been in bed at home for five months beforehand, and I was not allowed to go in and visit her. Of course, while she was in hospital, I never saw her. Mother received streptomycin and people were amazed at the speed of her recovery. She referred to Craig-y-nos as 'one big family' and seems to have enjoyed her stay there although she was unhappy about leaving her family for such a long time. However, she was very reluctant to talk about it and would reprimand me if I ever mentioned to anyone that she'd had TB. I got the impression that it was a taboo subject.

Ray Lewis died aged eighty-seven after enjoying excellent health after her discharge from Craig-y-nos.

Peter Gunn – A child with cystic fibrosis

My son, Christopher, was admitted to Craig-y-nos in the early 1950s, not with TB but with cystic fibrosis (an hereditary disease affecting mucus glands. The lungs may clog up with thick, sticky mucus and result in infections). He was in the Glass Conservatory (babies' ward). My wife, Joyce, and I were allowed to visit him every day, and the factory where we both worked adopted Craig-y-nos as its charity, sending toys at Christmas and Easter. We were told at first that Christopher had only three months to live. We prayed every night for him. My wife was praying that he would live and I was praying he would die, to be out of his pain.

The staff was wonderful. They adopted us. It was the most wonderful place he could ever have been with his health problems. We used to take him for walks in the grounds and his chest was wheezing constantly. He had such gentle ways, like his mother. Sister Powell adored my son. She used to take Christopher every day on the bus for a three-mile trip and back. Six weeks before he died, aged four, he said he didn't want to come home. In the day you would swear he was in a coma - very ill, couldn't walk - yet at night he was running up and down the cot singing *Jesus loves me*. After he died, Sister Powell wouldn't let him be taken to the morgue but had him put in her bed, and that's where we collected him.

There was a lack of psychological help for my wife and I after Christopher died. All she did was cry and cry. The trauma of the death of a child was not recognised in those days. I've still got Christopher's dummy, and a little ladder he had when he was about two-years-old, which my father, being a painter and builder, made. I still have the dressing gown he died in, and the table on which his coffin was placed. Even though we had a daughter, Lesley, our marriage broke up. Joyce re-married and I went into further education. I specialised in teaching people with brain-damage, combining my love of sport to introduce exercise for the handicapped. I found a new way to help progress people with learning disabilities towards social competence and a fuller life (for this pioneering work, Peter was awarded the MBE).

We planted a tree at Craig-y-nos in memory of Christopher. Joyce died last year and was buried in the same grave. They are together at last.

Staff stories

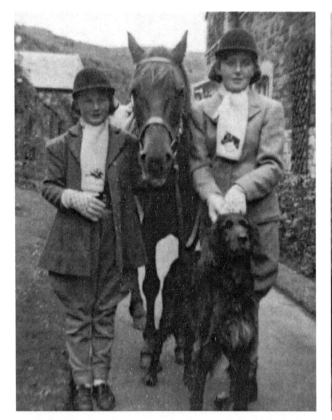

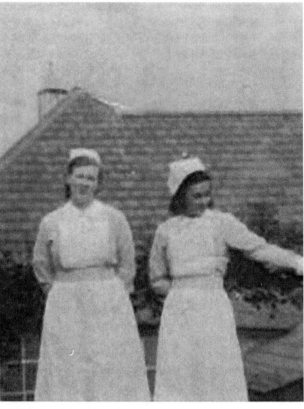

Mary (left) and Ruth with Paddy the Red Setter and pony. Courtesy Mary Sutton-Coulson.

Pat (left) with Mary Leo from Latvia. Courtesy Pat Davies.

Mary (right) and Ruth with Edgar, the head gardener, and Bonzo the Badger. Courtesy Mary Sutton-Coulson.

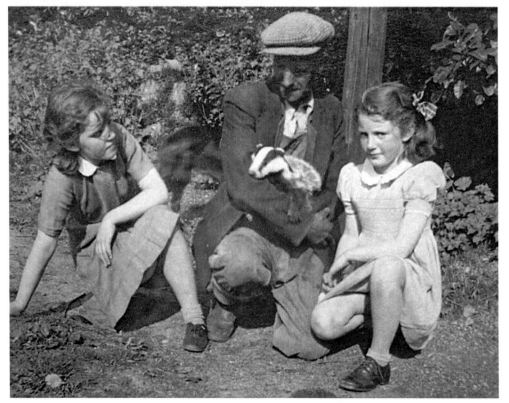

Pat Davies (Cornell) – Abandoned children

There was only one girl, Mary Morgan, and myself out on the balcony. It was mid-winter, 1944. We woke up one morning and Mary said, 'Can you move your legs?' I said, 'I don't know, I haven't tried yet.' 'Try to move them.' We couldn't. She said, 'Open your eyes.' And the snow was inches deep on the bottom of the bed. They couldn't open the balcony doors to get us in, so they had to send two porters round with a ladder to climb up onto the balcony to open the doors from the outside. Then they brought us in.

I had my eleventh birthday in Craig-y-nos and was only there for a year. It was the first time I'd been away from my mum and I cried a lot at first, but then I settled down quite well. We didn't have much schooling - the teachers came some days and not others. It was very difficult to catch up with schooling and I couldn't take the eleven-plus examination. I went to the secondary modern school and left at fifteen, but I always wanted to be a nurse. At seventeen, I went for an interview to Swansea General Hospital, and the Matron said, 'Oh no, my girl, I don't accept *anybody* who hasn't been to grammar school.' I felt really deflated but a few days later, in the *South Wales Evening Post,* there was an advert for nurses for Craig-y-nos. Matron Knox-Thomas, a fantastic woman, remembered me as a patient and gave me a job. That was 1951.

Well, we lived in the Nurses' Home and I had a room of my own. I remember most of the nurses who were there at the time - Glenys Davies, Peggy Taylor and Sally Jones. There were two Jean Evans's, Kathleen Fielding, Gwyneth Woodlake, and a German girl, Heather Schumann. We also had a Latvian nurse, Mary Leo, who'd been a displaced person. She'd originally come to work as a maid but Matron taught her English and she joined us as a nurse. She was very clever and also spoke fluent German and Polish. Night Sister used to wake us in the morning. She'd come into the Nurses' Home and knock on everybody's door. She'd put the light on at the back of your bed, and say, 'Seven o'clock, Nurse!' You had to get out of bed, strip it, get washed and dressed, and be in the dining room before half past seven, and then you went on duty. We'd change the patients' beds from the night to day covers, help with breakfasts, wash the patients, give out any medicines, and supervise those who were getting up. We'd make sure they were going for their walk. We went to lectures as well. Dr Hubbard occasionally gave lectures but most were given by the assistant matron, whose name was Rees (she was very small but wore platform shoes to make her look taller). Sister Outram, on Ward 4, was of the old school. She said, 'Right, you're going to learn everything I can teach you on this ward.' She was absolutely fantastic. I did gastric lavages and gave all the injections. Sister Jones, on Ward 1, couldn't give the streptomycin injections because it affected her very badly (she had become allergic to streptomycin – Glenys Davies was also badly affected). Sometimes, I'd be the only one on duty who *could* do them.

I felt that I could understand the patients more because I had been one myself. I could talk to them in a different way and I understood how frustrating it was to be tied in bed. If the children tried to get out of bed too often, they were put in restrainers. It was horrible but it was to make sure they did as they were told. One little girl, on a plaster bed, was going down for her operation and a number of us had to watch. It was performed by Mr (David) Rocyn-Jones (an orthopaedic surgeon who visited Craig-y-nos as a consultant. He was knighted in 1948). He took a fragment of bone from the pelvis and grafted it round her spine. He replaced part of her spine. It was fantastic. A couple of months later, one of the patients said, 'There's a little girl out here to speak to you.' It was the same child, and she said, 'Look, I'm walking.' As a nurse, you weren't supposed to show emotion and it's very difficult. I can remember the tears streaming down my face. I went outside and gave her a big hug. It was so wonderful - a little girl that couldn't remember walking. She'd have been nine or ten. There were a lot of orthopaedic operations on children with TB hip and Mr Rocyn-Jones would come to the hospital on certain days. Very often, children with TB hip were in plaster round their waist and down their leg. Sometimes the plaster would dig into their skin - into their bottom usually. I remember one little boy was crying one day and wouldn't tell me what was wrong. When we eventually turned him over, the plaster was cutting into his bottom. Dr Hubbard cut the plaster away and we had to use penicillin snuff (antibiotic powder) to fill the dent that it had made. Between supper time and before we went off duty, we'd do skin care to prevent pressure sores. We used methylated spirits and cream. Some of the children were on their backs for years, yet they never had pressure sores because Sister Jones and Sister Morgan insisted we treat them every day. Sometimes, however, patients would be admitted with pressure sores because they'd spent months in bed at home.

After Sister Outram (the dragon!) retired, Sister Roberts was in charge of Ward 4. She was a short, stubby little woman and always wore very strong perfume. I remember one instance when a young girl of fifteen was admitted. She was shown to her bed and after her mother had gone, Sister Roberts said, 'Would you take her for a bath to settle her in properly.' Sister came with me and went beserk because the girl had every type of infestation you could think of. She said, 'Go into the store room and get me some carbolic soap and two new nail brushes.' She put her in this bath and literally scrubbed her, and we also deloused her hair. Sister Roberts was very annoyed because she said that the girl was old enough to keep herself clean. That degree of infestation wasn't common. There were a lot of myths about TB and one stands out in my mind. When I was a patient we weren't allowed to have chewing gum. We were told that it was very bad for us. After one visiting day, a little girl on the balcony died and we were told it was because she'd eaten chewing gum.

Some children were literally dumped in Craig-y-nos, particularly those who'd survived TB meningitis and were deaf. Their parents didn't want to know and left them there. It was quite common and a number were adopted by local people. I remember 'Bubby', a local bus driver, adopting a child. There was one little girl on Ward 2 who'd been to Sully Hospital, Cardiff, to have a lung operation, and came to us afterwards. She was only about five or six. They tried to get in touch with the family but they didn't want to know. When she was fit enough to go into an orphanage, the women on Ward 1 rigged her out. They knitted cardigans and all sorts of things for her. Mr Jenkyn Evans, the dentist, always played Father Christmas. His daughter, Margaret, was admitted as a patient and I nursed her. She was about eighteen and could be very awkward at time but she survived (Margaret visited 'The Children of Craig-y-nos' exhibition in Swansea Museum).

We used to play badminton in the Patti Theatre with Dr Williams. We also had lots of shows, but listening to the Remembrance Day service from the Albert Hall, London, has always stuck in my mind. Matron Knox-Thomas insisted we listen and observe the two minutes silence (somebody told me that she'd lost her fiancé in the First World War). The children had to observe it too. When the hospital's first television – a tiny fourteen-inch set - was installed in the Patti Theatre, we'd watch the service. The Friends of the Hospital donated ward televisions for the Coronation in 1953. Matron made covers for them out of old red blankets and every night, when we switched off the televisions, we had to draw the covers like curtains. She was a very big lady and we always knew when she was coming into the ward. One day, we'd just finished the dinner round, and the pudding was Lyons ice cream – the little round blocks. The staff nurse had just popped one of these in her mouth, when suddenly we heard Matron approaching, and she swallowed it whole – icy cold – before going to greet her. On Ward 2, if I was on duty until eight o'clock, we'd have a singsong after the children had had their supper, the beds had been changed and we'd got the night rugs on. I'd take all the hair ribbons, wash them and bring them back into the ward to iron, and we'd sing. Everyone had their favourite songs. Ward 2 would always be chosen to sing for the hospital governors. We'd sing *Jerusalem* - 'Last night I lay sleeping, had a dream so fair, I stood in old Jerusalem beside the temple there …' When Harry Secombe performed in 'Jack and the Beanstalk' in the Patti Theatre at Christmas 1953, we had a patient on Ward 1 who was too ill to go to the performance and requested a special song. I went to ask him if he'd sing it and it was relayed to her over the loud speakers in the ward. She went home to die. Another Christmas, Matron had put mince pies and sherry for us in our sitting room and we'd all got into our pyjamas and dressing gowns when somebody had the bright idea that we'd go and sing carols. So, we went over to Dr Williams' house first, and it started snowing slightly. We sang carols outside and then we went up to Dr Hubbard's flat, and she was so thrilled. She'd been listening to a service coming from Austria. We used to have quite a lot of fun. I don't regret my time there.

I worked at Craig-y-nos until 1954, and the reason I left was that I'd met my future husband. We were getting married and the rule was, 'No married nurses'.

Pat has four children and is a great-grandmother. She lives in Coventry.

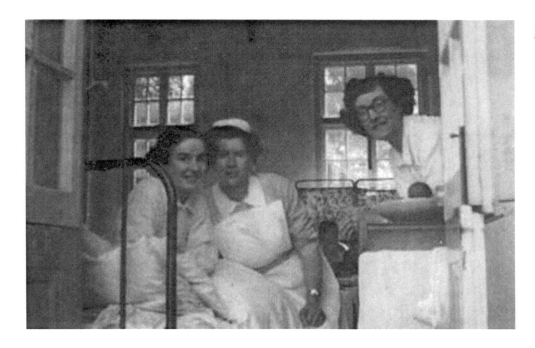

Pat (centre) with two of her patients, Amy Edwards and Mrs Northcote. Courtesy Pat Davies.

Some children were literally dumped in Craig-y-nos, particularly those who'd survived TB meningitis and were deaf...

...There was one little girl on Ward 2 who'd been to Sully Hospital, Cardiff, to have a lung operation, and came to us afterwards. She was only about five or six. They tried to get in touch with the family but they didn't want to know.

Pat Davies (Cornell)

Margaret Teresa Jones – part-time nurse

After hearing a broadcast appeal for part-time helpers at Craig-y-nos, and having several free hours every day when my husband was at work and my children at school, I applied for a position and was accepted. No previous nursing experience was necessary so I would begin as a very raw recruit, knowing nothing about hospitals except the little I had observed during the short period I had spent in one as a patient – only two weeks to be exact. Early the next Monday morning, after I had seen my children off to school, I went to the hospital to start my new work. I was taken to the sewing room and issued with a very starchy uniform and a small round cap which reminded me of Mrs Beeton. I was assigned to Ward 4, a new building, modern in style, which was built after Craig-y-nos had been converted from a country house into a hospital. The ward was bright and cheerful with large windows overlooking the lawns and the River Tawe which, in dry weather was a mere trickle but in the rainy season developed into a raging brown torrent, the roar of which could be heard clearly in the wards.

It was all quite strange and confusing at first and I had great difficulty in remembering the names of the twenty-four patients. Most of these were young girls but there were also several young married women. They were all very charming and friendly, and their gaiety and courage filled me with admiration. Their humour was all the more astonishing because many of them had to spend months, even years, away from their homes and children. They hardly ever grumbled and only an occasional one or two became depressed. Indeed, their cheerfulness was so infectious that they often cheered me up and made me see the lighter side of my several small troubles. I soon became accustomed to the unchanging routine of the ward. Every morning, the sweeping and dusting had to be done, beds made, flowers brought in from the bathroom where they were kept overnight, and everything tidied up in readiness for the doctors' daily visits. At ten o'clock the patients had what I think was meant to be 'elevenses' but which was called 'lunch'. After we had given this out and collected the cups, we got down to the serious business of blanket-bathing the bed-patients. This was very popular as it gave us a good excuse for having a nice long chat. Esconced in screens, we discussed everything under the sun – books, films, fashion, radio programmes, and our respective families. We soon knew all about each other and our children. My son's progress at school created enormous interest and when he passed an exam, he had a lovely surprise when a congratulatory telegram arrived, sent by the patients of the entire ward.

Some of the other jobs I had to do were filling hot-water bottles, helping to serve meals, washing combs and brushes, tidying lockers, changing library books, and of course, there was the inevitable bed-making. I have been at Craig-y-nos seven years now. They have slipped past with what seems incredible speed. I have seen hundreds of patients come in ill and go home cured. It gives me great satisfaction to know that I, in my humble and insignificant way, have helped to nurse so many of them back to health. I often think of them and I know they think of me too because every Christmas the largest number of my greeting cards come from ex-patients of Adelina Patti Hospital.

From an article in the South Wales Voice, 29 April 1955, sent to us by Margaret's son, Brian Jones.

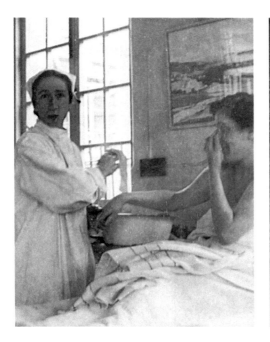 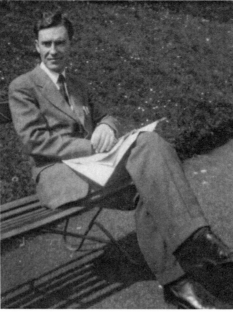

Morning wash. Margaret bed-bathing Rachel Davies (Morgan) on Ward 4. Courtesy Rachel Davies.

Dr Mulhall, a physician at Craig-y-nos from 1952-1985. Courtesy Sylvia Cottle.

Dr Patrick Plunkett Mulhall – The Swans

I went to Craig-y-nos first in 1952 to assist the Medical Superintendent at the time, Dr Ivor Williams, and I was there until 1985. I was based at Brecon. Patients in Craig-y-nos were getting on very well by 1952 because they were starting to get new drugs. It was a very strict regime: bed-rest - as much rest as possible - good food and fresh air. A lot of the children spent most of their time on the balconies. Before my time, they used to be left there in the rain, snow, everything. Of course, they were covered up but they had to endure that. There were also children in plaster casts for tuberculosis of bone joints and spines. Others had tuberculous glands of the neck. These were treated by ultra-violet rays and had a course of 'sun-ray' lamp treatment. Most of my work was with the adults, and they spent much of their time in bed but were gradually given graduated exercises to get them rehabilitated, and continued to walk outside the grounds. That's how they recovered, most of them.

There would be a monthly surgical session where a thoracic (chest) surgeon from Sully Hospital, Cardiff - Mr Dillwyn Thomas - performed minor operations such as cutting fibrous tissues (adhesions) in the pneumothorax (collapsed lung) cases. To collapse the lung, air would be inserted (through a needle) into the pleural space between the lung and the chest wall. Because of the disease, quite a number of the lung surfaces were adherent (stuck) to each other, and to the pleura on the chest wall, so they had to be separated to give a complete relaxation of the lung. It was collapsed down to its smallest size. Other patients - for example, those with lung cavities - were reviewed by the surgeon for possible surgery and transfer to the thoracic unit at Sully Hospital. Most of the people in Craig-y-nos had TB of the lungs. There were only a small number who had tuberculous bones and those were mainly children.

I don't recall any deaths in my time. The patients were selective in that the worst cases were transferred to surgical units and didn't come back. Perhaps some died after they went home, but I don't recall any sad cases of people dying in Craig-y-nos. Streptomycin and PAS (para-aminosalicylic acid) made a big difference. It changed the outlook completely for people who had diagnosed positive TB. Eventually, however, they found that people were becoming resistant to the new drugs. Then a new drug came in called isoniazid (discovered in 1952) and that was useful to help solve the problem of preventing patients developing resistance to the drugs. If the TB was uncontrolled by medication, it became apparent about six weeks after treatment, and if patients - particularly outpatients - took their drugs intermittently or not continuously, that could give rise to resistance very easily. It's the problem they have now in the third world. There were only a few members of staff, like Glenys Davies, who developed sensitivity to streptomycin. Gastric lavages were necessary to try and obtain some tuberculous bacilli (germs) in the gastric juices being swallowed. It was very difficult otherwise to get a specimen from the sputum. Some patients didn't have much sputum or they swallowed a lot of it. It was important to know whether the child was positive or negative so far as tuberculous bacilli was concerned. That also dictated what treatment they should need. It was not a very nice procedure at all for children (I wasn't involved in that) and these days they'd be a bit more refined. The techniques of doing that now are with simple tubes.

Dr Hubbard was a very strict doctor. Well, she didn't seem to have much feeling in one way, and then at other times she was very kind. She was a person who lived on her own in a flat up at the top of the building and I used to have my lunch with her in the dining-room adjoining to it once a week. She would never talk about her experiences, but she came from Vienna (she qualified MD in 1923 in Vienna), and got out before the Austrian Anschluss came into effect. She had polio as a child and used to limp around. She was a bit overweight and a formidable figure to these children. Dr Frank Wells was the first Medical Superintendent. He was there until 1927 when Dr Lizzie Robertson Clark became Superintendent. She was followed by Dr David Fenwick Jones who was, in turn, followed by Dr Ivor Williams. Dr Norman Jordan was a chest physician in Brecon but not at the Adelina Patti Hospital, unless he went there in a consultative capacity. He was a physician to the Welsh National Memorial Association, a post I inherited eventually. There were two secretaries, both ex-patients, in the office who ran the day-to-day administration and liaised so well with the patients for years. Ina Hopkins is deceased, but I still get Christmas cards from Euryl Thomas who lives near Craig-y-nos, in Abercrave.

The sanatorium originally had both male and female patients, but eventually the male patients were transferred to the North and South Wales sanatoria. TB male patients were difficult to control in the early days of a strict regime. One anecdote I heard was about two pals who asked permission from the Sister to go and see the swans in their allotted time of exercising. After several hours absence from the ward, the two lads arrived back looking the worse for wear, and on being asked where they had been, informed the Sister that they had been to see the 'Swans' (Swansea City Amateur Football Club) playing at their home venue in Swansea! Who can blame them?

Dr Mulhall lives in Brecon.

Ken Lewis – A family business

Ever since Adelina Patti's day, Craig-y-nos Castle has been a major source of employment for the area. When it became a hospital, a number of staff simply remained in the castle employment, with jobs passing down through families. Some jobs remained relatively unchanged, like gardening and general maintenance, and even today it is possible to trace employees whose relatives' had worked for Adelina Patti, like Edgar Davies, the head gardener. It's a close-knit community, intertwined with the life of the castle. Take my wife Ann, for example. Her grandfather was a boilerman, her father was the chauffeur, her uncle was Edgar Davies, and I also worked there as a stoker/boilerman. I'm eighty years-of-age now. There was a big campaign to keep the hospital open after the authorities wanted it closed as a TB sanatorium in 1958. The local community fought the proposed closure because it was the major source of employment in the area. Craig-y-nos remained open until 1986, first as a chest hospital then as a geriatric nursing home.

In my day, there were seven boilers for hot water dotted around the building, supplying water to the cast iron radiators. All the radiators were placed under the open windows and covered with metal grills. After the balconies were closed-in during the mid-1950s, radiators were put out there too. I can't recall fires in any of the wards although on very rare occasions, when the temperature was extremely low, Sister Morgan would agree to a small fire being lit in Ward 2. As for the staff, well, there was Christie, the head porter. I think he came from London, or maybe the north of England, I'm not sure. Victor Davies certainly came from London. He was in the army, and after demob got a job as a porter at Craig-y-nos. David John Richards, the hospital chauffeur, was his father-in-law. The chauffeur's job was to take patients to other hospitals, sometimes up to Welshpool or Llandrindod Wells. He worked there for twenty-five years

Sister Powell was the 'boss'. She was very fussy and would curry up to the doctors. I always remember her going into the grounds and picking daffodils, and taking them to Dr Williams' office and to Matron Knox-Thomas. She had to pass my window. She never took any to the children's wards. Matron Knox-Thomas was born and buried in Kendal. Once, a few of us went on a holiday and we called at Kendal to see the house where Matron Knox Thomas was born and the place where she was buried. At Christmas time, she used to roll her sleeves up and get in the kitchen to make the Christmas pudding for the whole hospital. She made all the male staff give sixpence each to put in the pudding. I used to take Dr Hubbard shopping to Brecon. She was very abrupt and hard, and the children didn't like her. She smoked like a trooper.

Craig-y-nos was, literally, one big happy family. We all worked together. I enjoyed working there and have lots of happy memories. I wish I had stayed there instead of going into the quarry.

Ken and Ann Lewis live in the village of Pen-y-cae, half a mile from Craig-y-nos.

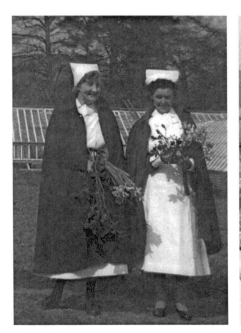
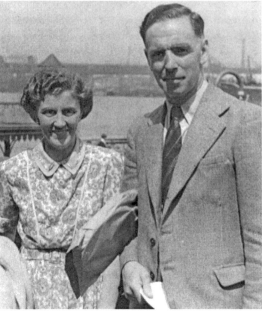

Sister Powell (left) with a bunch of daffodils, and Sister Lewis, who took Sister Morgan's place after her retirement. Courtesy Mary Watkins.

Dr Williams and his wife, Lyn. Courtesy Mary Sutton-Coulson.

Mary Sutton-Coulson (Williams) – Growing up in Craig-y-nos

My sister, Ruth, must have been six or seven when we went to Craig-y-nos in 1947, and I was three and a half. Mummy and Daddy (Dr Ivor Williams, the Medical Superintendent) met at Liverpool University and they both played hockey for Wales. My mother's parents were from Liverpool and they spoke Welsh. My mother, Lyn, spoke fluent Welsh. Daddy was born in Wrexham but their home was at Machynlleth (Powys). He spoke a bit of Welsh although he was much more anglicised. My parents married in 1936. They were very keen on sport and Daddy started a badminton club and the tennis club at Craig-y-nos. In the winter, after badminton, we'd go tobogganing in the moonlight on an army sledge down the hill opposite Craig-y-nos. One of the staff broke her leg one night by sticking it out as we went over a bump.

Craig-y-nos was the most amazing place for a child to live, although our house was dreadful for my mother because the kitchen was at the nearest end to the courtyard, the dining room was halfway down a corridor and our lounge was a square yellow block at the end. Then we had three storeys up to our attic bedroom, which for us was fantastic because we had a little link door into the Patti Theatre up in the eves. We used to watch all the performances given for the patients. Of course, if they were magic shows, we could see what was going on behind the scenes! Under the stage, which was linked to our basement, we had a table tennis table. Daddy was a very keen table tennis player. The floor in the Patti Theatre has a fascinating arrangement whereby it can be raised to a level with the stage so that it becomes a ballroom. We used to roller skate in the Theatre when the floor was flat, but when it's lowered it reveals the stage with the amazing painted fire screen of Madame Patti in her chariot, and a little orchestra pit. We had a croquet lawn where they now have the marquees (used for wedding receptions), and that was our garden. There were awful peacocks - one was called 'Jacko' - that used to preen themselves in the French windows and make such a noise in the morning.

Edgar, the head gardener, played a big part in helping us look after our ponies (Lady and Tosca) and also Matron's dog, Paddy, the Irish setter. What is now the Craig-y-nos Country Park car park was the most beautiful big vegetable garden. At the bottom right hand corner we had our stables and haystack. There were two large Victorian glasshouses against the wall by the lake, where Edgar grew peaches and lots of tomatoes. We were self-sufficient in fruit and vegetables but also had an area for chickens and ducks. We'd have about two dozen eggs a week and my mother would give spare eggs to Matron and others. One day Edgar's dog brought in two baby badgers. The mother must have been killed. One of the babies was dead but the other was alive so we looked after him and he lived in our stable. That was Bonzo. We would take him for walks on a lead but he used to bite Daddy! We also spent a lot of time messing about in the river and out in the boats on the lake.

We weren't really allowed near the children because of the chance of catching TB but we were allowed to go into the babies' ward (Glass Conservatory). The person I remember most and with great fondness is Sister Bessie Powell who was in charge of the babies' ward. After my sister went away to school, she was such a lovely lady and used to look after me if Mummy and Daddy were away. We'd pick mushrooms at six o'clock in the morning before I went to school. My father used to call her 'the menace'. He'd say, 'Have you and the menace been doing things again?' He had a very healthy respect for Bessie Powell. She was like his 'right-hand-man'. She lived in the 'Annexe' at the top of the walled vegetable garden with the other ward sisters. She had lost her fiancé in the First World War and never married (the same anecdote is told of Matron Mary Knox-Thomas). Bessie Powell came from Mountain Ash (Rhondda Cynon Taff) and bought a house there to retire but she was very, very sad to go back. We continued visiting her until she died. We also spent a lot of time in Matron Knox-Thomas' little flat if Mummy and Daddy were away. Harry Secombe came to the castle do a pantomime (1953), and I went and had tea with him and sat on his lap and had chocolate biscuits in Matron's flat. Ruth and I would sing on the hospital radio on Christmas Day for the patients. We always had to have our Christmas celebrations on Christmas Eve because Daddy carved the ward turkeys on Christmas Day. We had to be good little girls and have Christmas lunch with the sisters and Dr Hubbard. We'd have a laugh with her, I seem to remember. She was there always in the background.

Daddy liked being in charge of everything at Craig-y-nos and making things happen. We used to hold amazing Guy Fawke's parties every year, and he got terribly involved with the restoration of the Patti Theatre, bringing conservators from St Paul's Cathedral, London, to do all the gold leaf and restore the names of composers around the walls. He was also involved with the film about the life of Adelina Patti, starring Joan Sutherland and Paul Schofield. The BBC made a television programme about the hospital in the late 1950s showing Nurse Glenys Davies walking around the wards at night with a candle, against the background of Adelina Patti singing *There's no place like home*.

Nevertheless, it was a bit of a lonely life for me when my sister went to boarding school. Our friends were all the local farmers and there were only three neighbourhood farms - one either side of the hospital and the other at Dan-y-ogorf, near the caves. I'd spend my holidays up there sheep-shearing and feeding the baby lambs. We went to primary school at Pen-y-cae, and then the grammar school at Ystradgynlais, but that was seven miles away. I went to boarding school when I was twelve, to Abbots

Bromley School, Staffordshire. During the petrol crisis in the 1950s (the Suez Crisis, 1956) my parents didn't have enough petrol to drive Ruth and I to Staffordshire, so we went by train from Craig-y-nos Station, which involved five train changes! This was the little station at Penwyllt, which Adelina Patti built so that Edward VII could visit the castle (the station is closed but Patti's waiting room is still there).

My mother had trained as a biologist and botanist but there wasn't a school in the locality where she could teach these subjects, so she became very involved with various charities and Chairman of the Court in Ystradgynlais. My parents were very enthusiastic naturalists. I think they were early members of the conservation societies. They used to have us walking the Brecon Beacons and all around the Cray Reservoir. Every Sunday we'd go for walks. We would scramble up Craig-y-nos itself, that 'Rock of the Night', and pick lovely wild strawberries and blueberries. It was a very interesting childhood but at boarding school, we met up with people who lived in Leicestershire and Nottingham and Rugeley, who had a totally different sort of social childhood with all their parties and tennis clubs, etc. We'd spend quite a bit of time with them at weekends and holidays. Mummy and Daddy built a bungalow in Bronllys village, overlooking the Black Mountains, and spent their retirement there, which they absolutely loved. Daddy continued to play tennis until he was over seventy-five, and was passionate about his garden and his vegetables. He remained actively involved with the conservation of Wales. He died aged eighty-seven, in 1995, and my mother a few years earlier. In the end, Daddy did have a few minor strokes, so he became aphasic (loss of speech), which was very, very frustrating for him as he was such a sociable person.

Mary became a physiotherapist and lives in Hampshire. Ruth was a dentist and lives in Herefordshire.

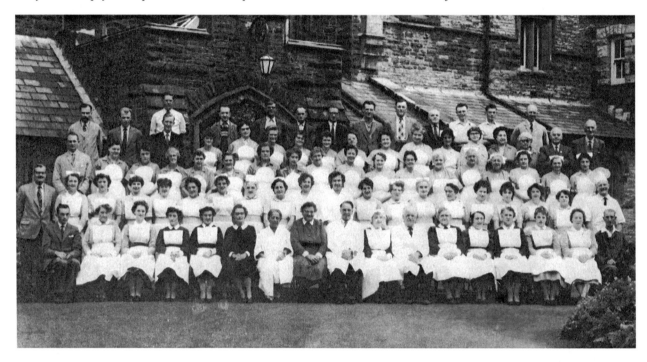

Front row *(left to right):* Doug Powell-engineer; nurses Meikle & Stella Price (Anthony), Sisters V Hodge & Betty Lewis, Miss Sullivan-Deputy Matron, Dr Pauline Huppert-Assistant Medical Officer, Matron Mary Knox-Thomas, Dr Ivor Williams-Medical Superintendent, Sister Bessie Powell, Jenkyn Evans-dentist, Sisters Gwyneth Lewis, Betty Lewis (Pugh) & Pearl Watkins, Nurses Sheila Price & Patey Taylor, Edgar Davies-Head Gardener.

Second row *(left to right):* John Barrows-engineer, Nurse Getta Hibbert, Joyce Cox-auxiliary, Student Nurses Glenys Waters & Beatrice Jones (Beamish), Auxiliaries Nancy Jones, Gwyneth Jones & Nancy Perrier, Medical Secretaries Ina Hopkins & Euryl Thomas, Student Nurse Margaret Williams, Auxiliaries Gladys Samuel, Lucy Thomas & Gladys Jones, Student Nurses Diane Hughes & Val James, Auxiliaries Hanna Williams & Mrs Bates, Gilbert Lake-chef.

Third row *(left to right):* John Heaven-Head Porter, Domestics Mrs Wellings, Gwen Bannister, Annie May Ellis, Hilda Lewis, Mrs Harvey, Mrs Jones, Mrs Dolly Jones & Mrs Turner, Margaret Heaven-Domestic Supervisor, Domestics Mrs Pugh, Marjorie Morris & Mrs Smith, Kitchen Domestics May Morris, Maggie Preace, Mrs Davies, Marion Williams & Mary Duvenas.

Fourth row *(left to right):* Porters Cliff Bannister & Alwyn Jones, John Cashmore-plumber, Mrs Donovan-domestic, Margaret Williams-auxiliary, Gwen Allexander-laundry domestic, Domestics Olive Morgan, Gwen Roberts, Mrs Powell, Dilys Gwilym & Mrs Rodrigues, Mrs Edgar Davies-Head Laundress, Sewing Mistresses Mary Emberton & Miss Daniels, Dai Richards-chauffeur, John Walters-painter.

Fifth row *(left to right):* Ken Lewis-boilerman/stoker, Sid Evans-porter, Gardeners Arthur Hales & Daniel John Price, Raymond Reece-painter, E Williams-carpenter, S Morris-gardener, Trevor Jones-painter, Gareth Morgan-porter, Elwyn Williams-gardener, Hubert Francis-porter.

Our gratitude to Glenys Jones (Davies) for naming most of the staff, and to Roy Harry for organising the research.

How could they treat
children the way they
did without any thought
or feeling? I am in my
seventies but the trauma
of those times still has
a profound effect on me.

Joan Wotton (Thomas)

Streptomycin and PAS
(para-aminosalicylic acid)
made a big difference.
It changed the outlook
completely for people
who had diagnosed
positive TB.

Dr Patrick Plunkett Mulhall

References

Introduction

1   *A Book Descriptive of Craig-y-nos Castle …* Estate Brochure, 1901. Brinn, David. 1988. *Adelina Patti: A Brief Account of Her Life.* Breacon Beacons National Park Committee. Cone, John Frederick. 1993. *Adelina Patti: Queen of Hearts.* Portland, Oregon: Amadeus Press. Klein, Herman. 1920 (reprinted 1978). *The Reign of Patti: Biography of the Great Lyric Soprano, Adelina Patti.* New York: Century Company; De Capo Press. Ley, Len. *Craig-y-nos Castle 1-10.* Powys Digital History Project: **http://history.powys.org.uk/history/ystrad/craig1.html** accessed 13 August 2007. Ley, Len. Personal research papers loaned to Carole Reeves.

2   Interview with Betty Lewis, 19 November 2007.

3   23rd Annual Report, Welsh National Memorial Association (WNMA), year ending 31 March 1935, p. 92. A1982/64, Box 13, Llyfrgell Genedlaethol Cymru/National Library of Wales (hereafter LGC).

4   Deeds and documents relating to the Adelina Patti Hospital. A1982/64, Box 15, LGC. Conveyance between WNMA and John Jones, 13 November 1931. A1982/64, Box 15, LGC.

5   33rd Annual Report, Welsh National Memorial Association (WNMA), year ending 31 March 1945, p. 2. A1982/64, Box 13, LGC.

6   Setting up of the Committee of Enquiry into the Anti-Tuberculosis Service in Wales, 1937, p. 15. A1982/64, Box 6, LGC.

7   Address by the President of the WNMA at the Annual Meeting of the Board of Governors, 25 June 1948. A1982/64, File 72 (ii), LGC.

8   Rating of hospitals, etc. A1982/64, Box 19, LGC.

9   Address by the President of the WNMA at the Annual Meeting of the Board of Governors, 25 June 1948. A1982/64, File 72 (ii), LGC.

10   Hershkovitz, Israel, Helen D Donoghue, David E Minnikin *et al.* 2008. 'Detection and molecular characterization of 9000-year-old Mycobacterium tuberculosis from a Neolithic settlement in the eastern Mediterranean.' *PLoS ONE* 3 (10): e3426. **www.plosone.org.**

11   Bryder, Linda. 1988. *Below the Magic Mountain: A Social History of Tuberculosis in Twentieth-century Britain.* Oxford: Clarendon Press. Dormandy, Thomas. 1999. *The White Death: A History of Tuberculosis.* London: Hambledon Press. Hardy, Anne. 2003. 'Reframing Disease: Changing Perceptions of Tuberculosis in England and Wales, 1938-70.' *Historical Research: the Bulletin of the Institute of Historical Research* 76: 535-56. Reeves, Carole. 2008. 'Tuberculosis in England since 1500.' In Joseph P Byrne (ed.), *Encylopedia of Pestilence, Pandemics, and Plagues.* Westport, CT: Greenwood Press, vol 2, pp. 709-12. Waddington, Keir. 2006. *The Bovine Scourge: Meat, Tuberculosis and Public Health, 1850-1914.* Rochester, NY: Boydell Press.

12   Deputation from Ystradgynlais Rural District Council about closure of Gellinudd and Adelina Patti Hospitals, 1962. Records of the Welsh Hospital Board, BD 18/2069, National Archives.

13   Consultations with local public bodies and organisations about hospital reorganisation in Swansea area: objections to closure of Adelina Patti Hospital, Craig-y-nos, 1968, 1969, Records of the Welsh Hospital Board, BD 18/2424 & BD/2425, National Archives.

14   Adelina Patti Hospital, estate brochure, 1986. WIAbNL 003328797, LGC.

15   Conry, Rosemary. 2002. *Flowers of the Fairest.* Dingle: Brandon Books.

16   Kelly, Susan. 2008. *Suffer the Little Children: Childhood Tuberculosis in the North of Ireland, 1865-1965.* PhD thesis, University of Ulster.

17   Connolly, Cynthia A. 2008. *Saving Sickly Children: The Tuberculosis Preventorium in American Life, 1909-1970.* New Brunswick, NJ: Rutgers University Press.

18   Bowlby, John *et al.* 1956. 'The Effects of Mother-child Separation: A Follow-up study.' *British Journal of Medical Psychology,* **29**: 211-247. Rosenbluth, Dina and John Bowlby. 1955. 'The social and psychological background of tuberculous children.' *British Medical Journal,* 1: 946-9. Bowlby, John. 1965 (second edition). *Child Care and the Growth of Love.* Harmondsworth: Penguin.

19 Rutter, Michael. 1972. *Maternal Deprivation Reassessed.* Harmondsworth: Penguin. Werner, Emmy E. 1984. *Child Care: Kith, Kin, and Hired Hands.* Baltimore: University Park Press.

20 Bryder, Linda. 1988. *Below the Magic Mountain. Op cit.,* pp. 210-12.

21 Davies, RPO *et al.* 1999. 'Historical Declines in Tuberculosis in England and Wales: Improving Social Conditions or Natural Selection?' *Vesalius,* 5: 25-29.

22 Setting up of the Committee of Enquiry into the Anti-Tuberculosis Service in Wales, 1937, p. 26. A1982/64, Box 6, LGC.

23 Adelina Patti Hospital school for handicapped children. School Inspectors' Report, 1936, p. 1. ED 224/23, National Archives.

24 Davies, Peter. 2005. 'An action plan for tuberculosis in England.' *Journal of the Royal Society of Medicine;* 98: 247-8.

25 Gandy, Matthew. 2008. 'Tuberculosis in the Contemporary World.' In Joseph P Byrne (ed.), *Encylopedia of Pestilence, Pandemics, and Plagues.* Westport, CT: Greenwood Press, vol 2, pp. 717-20. Gandy, Matthew and Alimuddin Zumla. 2003. *The Return of the White Plague: Global Poverty and the New Tuberculosis.* London: Verso.

Splendid isolation – Craig-y-nos, TB and treatment in the 1920s

1 Bryder, Linda. 1988. *Below the Magic Mountain. Op cit.,* p. 24.

2 Koch, Robert. 1906. 'The Nobel Lecture on how the fight against tuberculosis now stands.' *Lancet,* 1: 1449-1451.

3 WNMA Staff Journal no 2, 1921-4. A1982/64, Vol 63, LGC. WNMA Staff Register, 1913-37. A1982/64, Vol 66, LGC.

4 23rd Annual Report, Welsh National Memorial Association (WNMA), year ending 31 March 1935, p. 90. A1982/64, Box 13, LGC.

5 Interview with MT, 12 October 2007.

6 An open letter (undated but 1927) from FJ Alban, General Secretary, WNMA. A1982/64, Box 15, LGC.

7 Letter from William Leyson of Neath to FJ Alban, WNMA, Cardiff, 19 August 1927. Lease of shooting and fishing rights at Adelina Patti Hospital to Thomas J Davies. A1982/64, Box 15, LGC.

8 WNMA Accounts for the year ended March 31, 1934. A1982/64, Box 13, LGC.

9 List of equipment purchased for Adelina Patti Hospital, passed by the WNMA Finance Committee, 13 July 1922. A1982/64, Box 3, LGC.

Instant sunshine – Craig-y-nos, TB and treatment in the 1930s

1 Rating of hospitals, etc. A1982/64, Box 19, LGC.

2 Adelina Patti Hospital school for handicapped children. School Inspectors' Report, 1936, p. 1. ED 224/23, National Archives.

3 'Immediate steps to cope with waiting lists'. A1982/64, Box 7, LGC.

4 'The King Edward VII Welsh National Memorial Association for the Prevention, Treatment and Abolition of Tuberculosis'. WNMA, *c.*1932. A1982/64, File 72 (i), LGC.

5 23rd Annual Report, Welsh National Memorial Association (WNMA), year ending 31 March 1935, page 89. A1982/64, Box 13, LGC.

6 Kayne, G Gregory. 1934. 'A note on the study of pulmonary tuberculosis in infants and children' *British Medical Journal,* 3 March: 1-5. A1982/64, Box 9, LGC. Central Tuberculosis Laboratory, Welsh National School of Medicine, Newport Road, Cardiff. A1982/64, File 72 (i), LGC.

7 WNMA Staff Register, 1913-37. A1982/64, Vol 66, LGC.

8 Information from Amy Evans' daughter, Moira Paterson.

9 23rd WNMA Annual Report, year ending 31 March 1935, p. 16. A1982/64, Box 13, LGC. Adelina Patti Hospital House Committee, 22 May 1939, note 2527. A1982/64, Box 7, LGC. WNMA Report of Committee of Inquiry into the Anti-Tuberculosis Service in Wales and Monmouthshire. Recommendations and Opinions of Committee to the Minister of Health, 17 March 1939. A1982/64, Box 7, LGC. WNMA Special Committee, Cardiff, April 21, 1939, p. 1546. In Report of the Committee of Enquiry (set up by the Minister of Health) into the Anti-Tuberculosis Service in Wales and Monmouthshire, 1937. A1982/64, Box 7, LGC.

10 Swansea County Council to Ministry of Health, 16 August 1935. *Western Mail,* 2 October 1935. Welsh Board of Health. MH96/1008, National Archives.

11 The Association's 5-year estimates 1937-42 relating to Adelina Patti Hospital, p. 271. A1982/64, Box 7, LGC. WNMA Schedule of Capital and Extraordinary Expenditure proposed or contemplated during the above period (1937-1942). Issued January 1937. A1982/64, Box 13, LGC. Scheme to be made by the Minister of Health under Section 102 (3) of the Local Government Act, 1929, for the third fixed grant period, 1937-1942. A1982/64, Box 13, LGC.

12 Changes in medical staff, confidential memorandum. A1982/64, Box 23, LGC. Dr Ivor Williams, personal staff file. A1982/64, Box 23, LGC.

13 WNMA Staff Register, 1913-37. A1982/64, Vol 66, LGC.

14 WNMA Staff Register, 1913-37. A1982/64, Vol 66, LGC.

15 Setting up of the Committee of Enquiry into the Anti-Tuberculosis Service in Wales, 1937. A1982/64, Box 6, LGC.

16 Death-rates from tuberculosis in administrative counties and county boroughs, England and Wales, 1931. In National Association for the Prevention of Tuberculosis (NAPT) Council Report, 1932. In Bryder, Linda. 1988. *Below the Magic Mountain. Op. cit.,* p. 12.

17 Setting up of the Committee of Enquiry into the Anti-Tuberculosis Service in Wales, 1937. A1982/64, Box 6, LGC.

18 33rd WNMA Annual Report, year ending 31 March 1945, p.51. A1982/64, Box 13, LGC.

19 23rd WNMA Annual Report, year ending 31 March 1935, p. 88. A1982/64, Box 13, LGC.

20 Correspondence between WNMA and Marmite Food Extract Company, 1938. A1982/64, File 20, LGC.

Magic bullets – Craig-y-nos, TB and treatment in the 1940s

1 WNMA detailed estimate for the year ending March 31, 1942. A1982/64, Box 13, LCG. Dr Ivor Williams, personal staff file. A1982/64, Box 23, LGC.

2 33rd WNMA Annual Report, year ending 31 March 1945, p. 28. A1982/64, Box 13, LGC.

3 Adelina Patti Hospital School log book, 1947-1972. Powys Archives.

4 Minutes of a Meeting of the Finance Committee, 8 April 1948. A1982/64, Box 9, LGC.

5 33rd WNMA Annual Report, year ending 31 March 1945, p. 51. A1982/64, Box 13, LGC.

6 33rd WNMA Annual Report, year ending 31 March 1945, pp. 34, 54. A1982/64, Box 13, LGC.

7 Adelina Patti Hospital school for handicapped children. School Inspectors' Report, 1944-45, p. 1. ED 224/23, National Archives.

8 General Nursing Council for England and Wales: Education: Nurse training schools. Report on visit to Adelina Patti Hospital, 8 December 1945. DT 35/231, National Archives.

9 Adelina Patti Hospital school for handicapped children. School Inspectors' Report, 1944-45, p. 1. ED 224/23, National Archives.

10 HO 405/22008, National Archives.

11 Weindling, Paul. 2006. 'Medical Refugees in Wales 1930s-50s.' In Pamela Michael and Charles Webster (eds.), *Health and Society in Twentieth Century Wales.* Cardiff: University of Wales Press, pp. 183-200.

12 Personal communication, 22 April 2008.

13 Adelina Patti Hospital school for handicapped children. School Inspectors' Report, 1953, p. 1. ED 224/23, National Archives.

14 Marshall, Geoffrey *et al.* 1948. 'Streptomycin Treatment of Pulmonary Tuberculosis: A Medical Research Council Investigation.' *British Medical Journal*; **2**: 769-82. Crofton, John. 2004. 'The MRC Randomised Trial of Streptomycin and its Legacy: A View from the Clinical Front Line.' The James Lind Library (www.jameslindlibrary.org)

15 Dr Thomas Francis Jarman, personal staff file. A1982/64, Box 22, LGC.

16 Script from 'Searchlight on TB', BBC Welsh Home Service, transmitted Tuesday 14 June 1949, 9.35-10.05 pm. A1982/64, Box 9, LGC.

Emotional deprivation – Craig-y-nos, TB and treatment in the 1950s

1   General Nursing Council for England and Wales: Education: Hospital Inspectors' Reports and Papers. Adelina Patti Hospital. DT 33/2035, National Archives.

2   Adelina Patti Hospital school for handicapped children. School Inspectors' Report 1953, pp. 1-2. ED 224/23, National Archives.

3   Adelina Patti Hospital school for handicapped children. School Inspectors' Report 1958. ED 224/23, National Archives.

4   Walker-Smth, J A. 1997. 'Children in hospital'. In Irvine Loudon (ed.), *Western Medicine*. Oxford: Oxford University Press, pp. 221-31.

5   Bowlby, John. 1951. *Maternal care and mental health*. Geneva: World Health Organization, Monograph Series, no 2. Bowlby, John. 1953. 'Some pathological processes set in train by early mother-child separation.' *Journal of Mental Science*, **99**: 265-72. Bowlby, John. 1965 (second edition). *Child Care and the Growth of Love*. Harmondsworth: Penguin. Bowlby, John *et al*. 1956. 'The Effects of Mother-child Separation: A Follow-up study.' *British Journal of Medical Psychology*, **29**: 211-247. Dina Rosenbluth and John Bowlby. 1955. 'The social and psychological background of tuberculous children.' *British Medical Journal*, 1: 946-9.

6   Drolet, Godias J and Anthony M Lowell. 1962. 'Tuberculosis mortality among children: the last stage. A statistical review of the 1950-1959 decade in Canada, the United States, England and Wales, and France.' *Chest* **42**: 364-71.

7   Tuberculosis Chemotherapy Centre, Madras. 1959. 'A concurrent comparison of isoniazid plus PAS with sanatorium treatment of pulmonary tuberculosis in South India.' *Bulletin of the World Health Organization* **23**: 535-85.

8   Memo dated 16 June 1959, Department of Education. ED 224/23, National Archives.

Alphabetical list of people who have contributed stories and / or photographs to this project. Those in italics appear in this book.

Baglan, Beth Rees
Baker, Sue
Barker, Jeanette
Barnes (Watkins), Delphine
Barry (O'Shea), Molly
Bartlett (Griffiths), Renée
Bater, Brenda
Batts, John
Bebell, Harry
Beechey, Molly
Bennett (Snell), May
Beynon, Haydn
Beynon, Roger Wyn
Blake, Ann
Blake (Howells), Margaret
Blatchford (Hoyles), Myfanwy
Blewett (Paris), Vera
Booth, David
Booth, John
Bowen (Hill), Pamela
Bowen, Shirley
Boyce (Havard), Caroline
Brace (Thomas), Megan
Branson, Suzy
Brent (Price), Valerie
Bufton, Milwyn
Clements (Berry), Jean
Collins (Coughlan), Joan
Cottrill (Gordon), Mary
Cottle (Price), Sylvia
Creighton (Rees), Catherine Ann
Davies, Alcwyn
Davies, Gerwyn
Davies (Bevan), June
Davies (Evans), Lynette
Davies (Maddock), Margaret
Davies (Morris), Mary
Davies (Murphy), Mary
Davies, Nan
Davies (Cornell), Pat
Davies (Morgan), Rachel
Davies (Harley), Rosemary
Davies, Will
Dodd, Vanessa
Ealston, Glennis
Evans, Debbie
Evans, Gwanwyn
Evans (Wakeham), Jeanette
Evans (Allsopp), Robert
Evans, Tegan
Evans, Vernon
Farley, Doreen

Floyd (Williams), Sylvia
Forsey, Kaye
Friend (Jenkins), Mari
Gardiner, Ann
Gardiner, Peter
Gardiner (Gammon), Winnie
Gibbons (Hill), Eileen
Glass (Whitelock), Anna
Gordon, Mary
Greenow, Ruth
Gunn, Peter
Hamer (Osmond), Pamela
Hansen, Sandy
Harris, Haydn
Harris (Edwards), Mair
Harry, Roy
Hayes, Soren
Herbert, Douglas
Hixon, Sonia
Hopkins (Phillips), Jean
Hughes (Davies), Carol
Hunt, Terry
Hybert (Mogridge), Pat
Ireland (Jones), Mary
Isaac, Thomas Edward
Jakes, Betty
Jones, Brian
Jones (Thomas), Christine
Jones (Morgan), Gaynor
Jones, Glanville
Jones (Davies), Glenys
Jones, Hilary
Jones, Margaret Teresa
Jones, Non
Jones (Morris), Patricia
Jones (Dobson), Peggy
Jordan, Sybil
Joseph, Olive Pamela
Lewis, Ann
Lewis, Beryl
Lewis, Betty
Lewis, Ken
Lewis (Pearce), Norma
Lewis, Phil
Ley, Len
Lowe, Glynne
McNie, James
Michael, Pat
Morgan, Alan
Morgan, Geraint
Moore (Peckham), Sylvia
Morris, Ann
Mortali, Gaye
Mulhall, Patrick Plunkett
Mullen, Cynthia
Mullins, Royston
Munson (Lewis), Lotte
Nelson, John
O'Byrne (Mathoulin), Pat
O'Connell (Paines), Barbara
Oltersdorf (Lewis), Dulcie

Owen, Avril
Parle, Stephen
Paterson, Moira
Perkins, Peter Leslie Stacey
Perrott, David
Perry (Bennett), Christine
Perry, Larry
Peters (Williams), Ann
Philibosian (Hopkins), Marlene
Poole (Bebell), Thelma
Powell, Maureen
Price, Aubrey
Price, John
Pridding, James Albert
Pugh (Hunt), Rose
Pugh, Stephen
Pye (Dommett), Barbara
Rees (Thomas), Myra Elizabeth
Reeves, Diana
Rich, Margaret
Richard, Alan
Richards (Rowlands), Beryl
Richards, Brian
Richards (Berry), Jean
Richards (Driscoll), Mary
Roberts, Eurwen
Robson, Bridget
Rogers, Wendy
Ronan, Bridie
Rowlands, Clive
Sambrook, Byron
Shaw (Rumsey), Ann
Slater (Davies), Mary
Smallwood, Richard
Smith (Allsopp), Judy
Stead, Royden
Sutton-Coulson (Williams), Mary
Tayler, Jane
Telesford, Edward
Thomas, Annette
Thomas (Dowdle), Betty
Thomas, Edward Ellis
Thomas, Euryl
Thomas, Gwyn
Thomas, Margaret
Thomas (Hughes Richards), Margaret
Thomas (John), Marian
Thomas (Phillips), Megan
Thomas (Elson), Sandra
Thornton (Davies), Christine
Tizzard (Jones), Peggy
Turner (Gleed), Sue
Wagstaffe, Peter
Walton, Glennis
Watkins (Williams), Mary
Whitlock, Sharon
Williams (Morgan), Glenys
Williams, Neville
Williams (Llewellyn), Valerie
Wotton (Thomas), Joan
Wyke, Gareth

CPSIA information can be obtained at www.ICGtesting.com
Printed in the USA
LVOW130241250212

270334LV00001B/71/P